ALSO BY CONSTANCE SANTEGO

FICTION
(Novels based on actual events)
The Nine Spiritual Gifts Series:
Journey of a Soul

NONFICTION
The Intuitive Life, A Guide to Self-Knowledge and Healing through Psychic Development Second Edition

Fairy Tales, Dreams and Reality... Where Are You On Your Path? Second Edition

Your Persona... The Mask You Wear

Angelic Lifestyle, A Vibrant Lifestyle

Archangel Michael's Soul Retrieval Guide

SECRETS OF A HEALER, SERIES:

Magic Of Aromatherapy (Vol I)
Magic Of Reflexology (Vol II)
Magic Of The Gifts (Vol III)
Magic Of Muscle Testing (Vol IV)
Magic Of Iridology (Vol V)
Magic Of Massage (Vol VI)
Magic Of Hypnotherapy (Vol VII)
Magic Of Reiki (Vol VIII)

Angelic Lifestyle 42-Day Energy Cleanse
Copyright © 2020 by Constance Santego.

Copy Editor and Interior Design: Constance Santego
Book Layout: ©2017 BookDesignTemplates.com
Cover Design: Canva

Ordering Information:
Quantity sales. Special discounts are available on quantity purchases by corporations, associations, and others. For details, contact the "Special Sales Department" at the address above.

Trade paperback ISBN: 978-1-7770818-3-6
eBook ISBN 978-1-7770818-4-3
Cover: Canva
Created and published In Canada. Printed and bound in the United States of America

First Edition
Published by Maximillian Enterprises
Kelowna, BC
Canada
www.constancesantego.ca

Angelic Lifestyle's

42 - Day
Energy Cleanse

Method & Recipe Book

Easy recipes and essential information for A Vibrant Lifestyle
From a Grand Reiki Master
Constance Santego

Maximillian Enterprises
Kelowna, BC

Companion Book

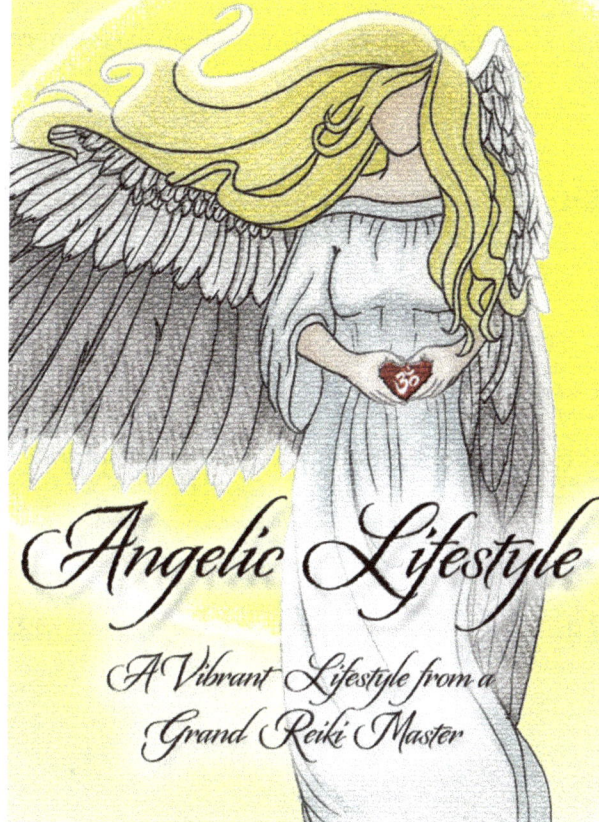

Constance Santego

Angelic Lifestyle

A Vibrant Lifestyle from a
Grand Reiki Master

Dedication

To All My Energy & Natural Health Teachers

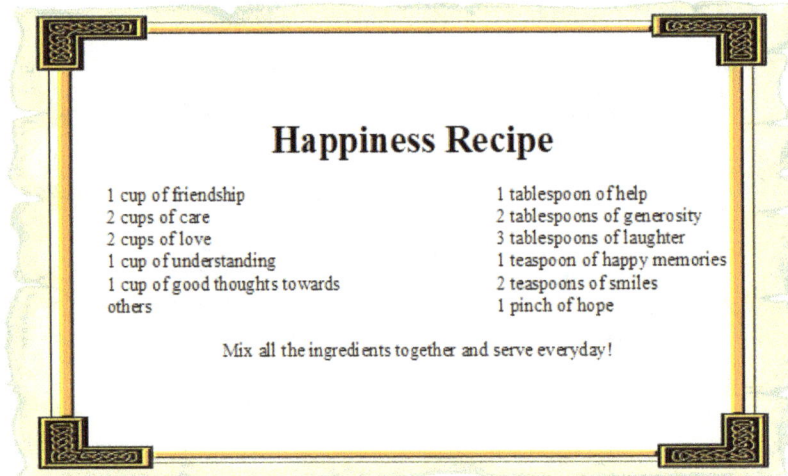

Happiness Recipe

1 cup of friendship
2 cups of care
2 cups of love
1 cup of understanding
1 cup of good thoughts towards others

1 tablespoon of help
2 tablespoons of generosity
3 tablespoons of laughter
1 teaspoon of happy memories
2 teaspoons of smiles
1 pinch of hope

Mix all the ingredients together and serve everyday!

Your Body Is Your Temple,
too bad the mind forgets that sometimes!

–Constance Santego

Angelic Lifestyle's

42 - Day

Energy Cleanse

Contents

Preface

In the bible 'The Gift of Healing' is granted from Spirit and is one of the nine spiritual gifts granted. Self-healing is as important as healing others, some may say even more so. If you are not healthy how can you help others? On an airplane, the flight attendant tells you to put on your air mask first, then to help others.

After reading, 'Angelic Lifestyle, A Vibrant Lifestyle,' the first book in this series, you will have understood the importance of Homeostasis (Balance) in your body, mind, and soul. In Quantum Medicine it is your Physical, Vital, Mental, Supramental, and Blissful Body that you are balancing.

In this book, 'Angelic Lifestyle's 42-Day Energy Cleanse Method & Recipe Book' you will be able to take your new knowledge and apply it while you are following the 42-Day Cleanse. The Angelic Lifestyle is a wonderful way to empower your life.

Shift happens... Create Magic!

Enjoy changing your life one day at a time!
Constance

Note to Reader

THIS IS NOT A DIET!!!
The Angelic Lifestyle is not to replace modern medicine. It is solely to gain vitality back into your body, mind, and soul.

The Angelic Lifestyle's diet portion follows the Canadian Food Guide.

The understanding of Integrated Medicine is that **we play** a significant role in taking care of our own health. Knowing what we put into our bodies, how hard we work our bodies, the stress level we allow into our life, and the positive or negative energy we attract around us all play a role in our wellbeing. The purpose of this Angelic Lifestyle is to rid our body, mind, and soul of negative energy and bring in more positive vitality.

Shift happens...Create magic!

The Goal

Simply to gain vitality and bring your wishes, wants, dreams, and desires into reality!

You cannot buy more clothes if your closet is jammed packed. You will need to cleanse the space to make more room for the new ones.

Same rule goes for your body, mind, and soul!

xxiv CONSTANCE SANTEGO

Part One

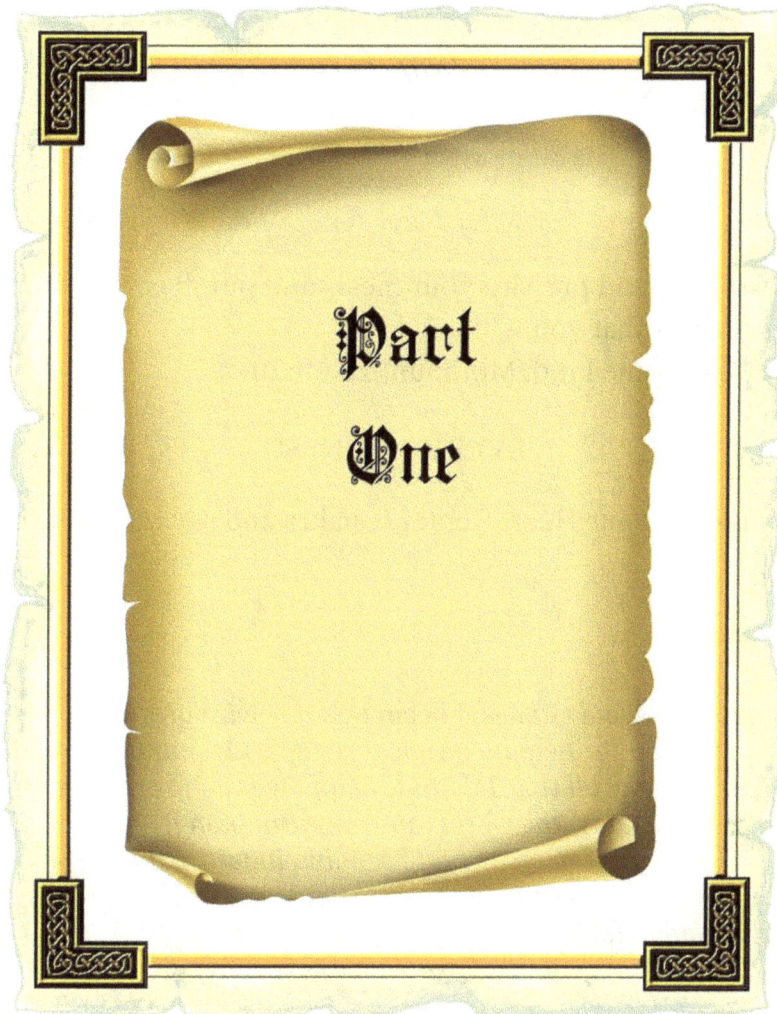

Angelic Lifestyle's 42-Day Energy Cleanse

Day One

Today's Goal

- Read Part Two, plan and prepare your meals and purchase the food, vitamins, minerals, and drinks that you will need.
- Add in exercise of some kind. Minimum 10 minutes.

EVERY MORNING

1st Put your hands over your Heart Center/Chakra and say out loud this morning blessing.

Morning Blessing

> *"I call upon my Angels and Guides, I begin this day with gratitude, love, and abundance. I would like to thank you for helping me cleanse my body, mind, and soul during the night. I will do my best to make all that I do today empowering for my life's journey and purpose. God bless this day, the world, and everything on it. As I take my next breath, I am envisioning healing green energy and sending it out to anyone who needs it, including myself. I ask and give you permission to help guide me throughout my day...*
> *Love and Light, Namaste"*

2nd Do at least one round of the Eight Essential Standing Exercises. Keeping a flexible body is essential to aging (full technique is explained in the Angelic Lifestyle's Vibrant Lifestyle Book).

Sometime during the day Go for a walk or some other kind of fitness (minimum 10 minutes). Cleaning the house, gardening, or shoveling the snow counts.

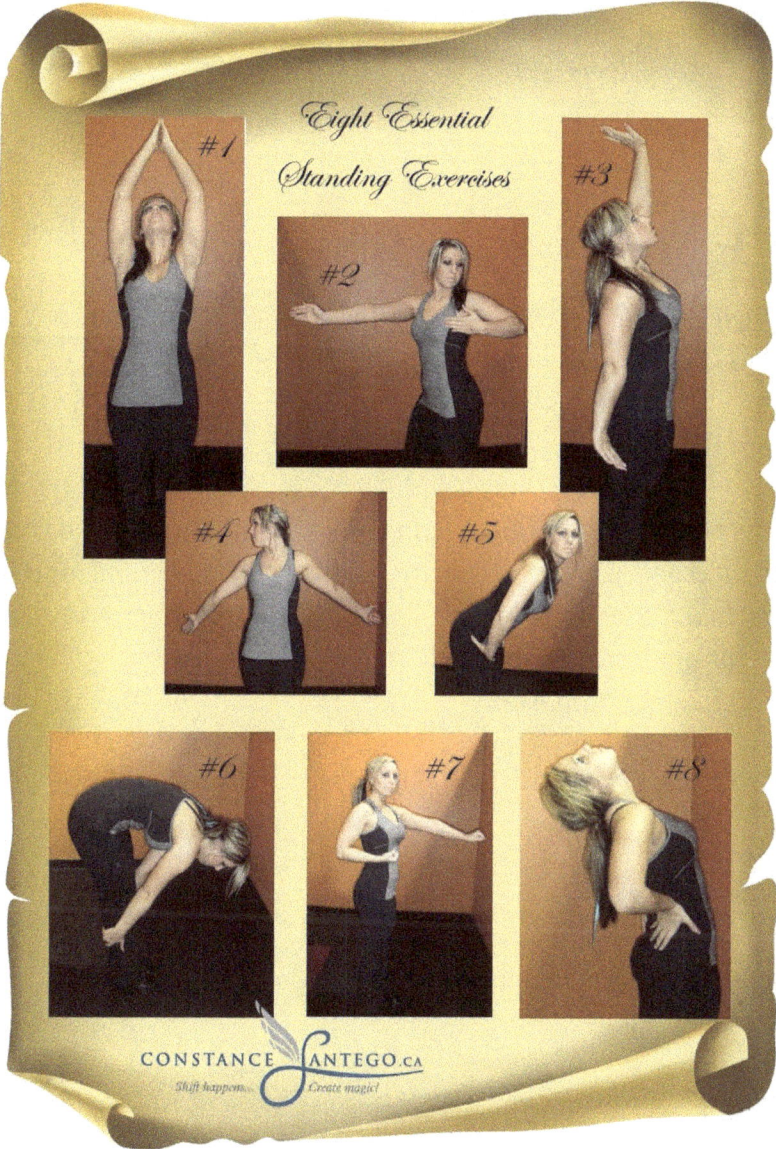

Eight Essential Standing Exercises

#1 #2 #3 #4 #5 #6 #7 #8

CONSTANCE SANTEGO.CA
Shift happens... Create magic!

3rd Before anything enters your mouth, bless the item(s) by thinking or saying,

Choice the appropriate one:
"Bless this food and drink."
"Bless this food."
"Bless this drink."

Today, fulfill the Goal

➤ Do steps 1 -3 and plan your meals (part three has recipe ideas).

Bedtime

42-Day activation – Say this tonight to activate healing, "I am truly blessed. I wish my Angels and Guides good night, every night, and give you permission to cleanse my body, mind, and soul as you see fit. Knowing that you are taking the energy to be cleansed and replacing it for my highest good. I give you permission for any excess to be gifted to the Celestial World to be used as needed there or on Earth. Love and Light, Namaste."

EVERY EVENING BEFORE BED

Evening Blessing
Put your hands over your Heart Center/Chakra and say this evening blessing out loud.

"Thank you to my Angels and Guides for helping me towards fulfilling my life's lessons, purpose, and journey."

Day Two

Today's Goal

- Learn & do a self-Reiki treatment

MORNING

1st Put your hands over your Heart Center/Chakra and say out loud the morning blessing.

2nd Do at least one round of the Eight Essential Standing Exercises.

3rd Before anything enters your mouth, bless the item(s). Follow your days plan for today's food and drink intake.

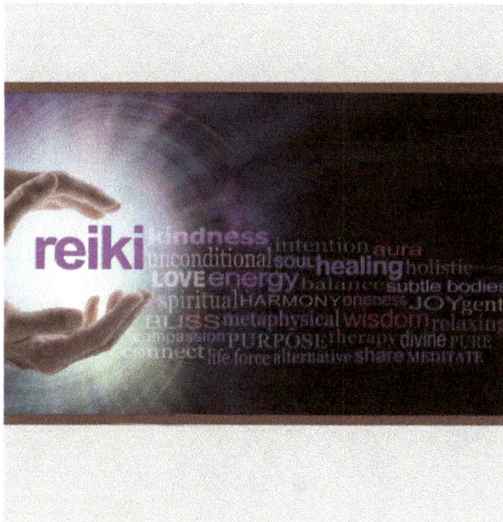

NEW TODAY 4th Do self-Reiki,

➤ If you do not already have Level 1 Reiki, go to
o My Constance Santego Website (www.constancesantego.ca),
▪ Connie's Inspirations,
▪ Workshops,
▪ Reiki

Today, Fulfill the Goal

> ➢ Even if all you can do today is listen to the Level 1 Reiki Video, do that at least.
> ➢ Do a self-Reiki treatment on yourself

Bedtime

Evening Blessing
Put your hands over your Heart Center/Chakra and say this evening blessing out loud.

"Thank you to my Angels and Guides for helping me towards fulfilling my life's lessons, purpose, and journey."

Day Three

Today's Goal

- Add in the Quick Fix Procedure

MORNING

1ˢᵗ Put your hands over your Heart Center/Chakra and say out loud the morning blessing.

2ⁿᵈ Do at least one round of the Eight Essential Standing Exercise

And sometime during the day go for a walk or some other kind of fitness (minimum 10 minutes).

3ʳᵈ Before anything enters your mouth, bless the item(s). Follow your days plan for today's food and drink intake.

4ᵗʰ Do self-Reiki, (minimum 1 minute).

NEW Today -5ᵗʰ

Do the 'Quick Fix' procedure to balance all your meridians.

QUICK FIX

For further information read,
'Secrets of a Healer – Magic of Muscle Testing.' (Rub all the points)

Muscle Testing - Quick Fix

1) Ask client to sense his body's area(s) of pain. On a scale of 1-10, 10 being major pain, ask the client to tell you his level.
2) Lightly rub or have client rub all the front and back Neuro-lymphatic points.
3) Have client take a deep breath and re-sense his level of pain.
4) If the pain has not come down to 0, redo the "quick fix" sequence.
5) If pain level does not come to 0 the second time, the client may need to have a chiropractic adjustment or need a different type of treatment, or you may try to relax/quiet individual muscles.

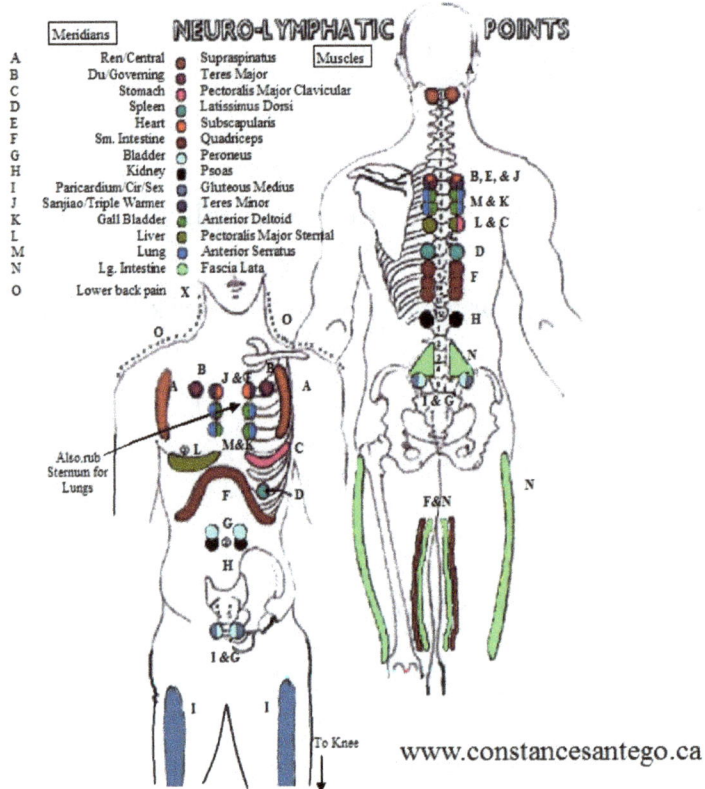

NEURO-LYMPHATIC POINTS

	Meridians		Muscles
A	Ren/Central		Supraspinatus
B	Du/Governing		Teres Major
C	Stomach		Pectoralis Major Clavicular
D	Spleen		Latissimus Dorsi
E	Heart		Subscapularis
F	Sm. Intestine		Quadriceps
G	Bladder		Peroneus
H	Kidney		Psoas
I	Paricardium/Cir/Sex		Gluteous Medius
J	Sanjiao/Triple Warmer		Teres Minor
K	Gall Bladder		Anterior Deltoid
L	Liver		Pectoralis Major Sternal
M	Lung		Anterior Serratus
N	Lg. Intestine		Fascia Lata
O	Lower back pain	X	

Also rub Sternum for Lungs

To Knee

www.constancesantego.ca

Today, Fulfill the Goal

> ➤ Rub all the colored areas (front & back) on your body, from the 'Quick Fix' chart. Knowing that each time you rub these spots you are balancing your body, mind, and soul, becoming healthier, and more vibrant!

Bedtime

Evening Blessing
Put your hands over your Heart Center/Chakra and say this evening blessing out loud.

"Thank you to my Angels and Guides for helping me towards fulfilling my life's lessons, purpose, and journey."

Day Four

Today's Goal

- Add in Meditation

MORNING

1st Put your hands over your Heart Center/Chakra and say out loud the morning blessing.

2nd Do at least one round of the Eight Essential Standing Exercise

And sometime during the day go for a walk or some other kind of fitness (minimum 10 minutes).

3rd Before anything enters your mouth, bless the item(s). Follow your days plan for today's food and drink intake.

4th Do self-Reiki, (minimum 1 minute).

5th Do the 'Quick Fix' Procedure.

NEW Today 6th

> A) Once a week do this Negative Energy Clearing Meditation (Go to Constance Santego YouTube Channel and listen to the meditation or have someone read this to you.).

NEGATIVE ENERGY &
CHAKRA CLEARING MEDITATION

1. Make yourself comfortable in a chair or lie down
2. When you are ready close your eyes
3. Imagine your *Root Chakra* (the lowest point of your torso)
   a. Imagine a <u>red</u> flower opening up...any type of flower will do,
   b. Imagine that there are cords attached to you here. The Huna or Kundalini called these 'aka' cords.
   c. Now imagine all of these cords that are not yours being released lovingly to whomever they belong to, and all of yours coming back to you.
   d. You can imagine releasing them like you would a cable from your computer or phone,
   e. Great, now wait a few moments while this chakra is being cleansed
   f. If there are too many to release right now, know that you can always come back to this chakra again later,
   g. Take a deep breath,
   h. Imagine that there is a clear bubble formed over top of this area for protection.
4. Imagine your *Sacral or Sex Chakra* (the area between your root and belly button).
   a. Imagine an <u>orange</u> flower opening...
   b. Imagine these aka cords that are attached to you here,
   c. Again, imagine all of these cords that are not yours being released lovingly to whomever they belong to and all of yours coming back to you,
   d. And wait again a few moments while this chakra is being cleansed,
   e. Take a deep breath,

f. Imagine a clear bubble over top of this area for protection.

5. Now, imagine your *Solar Plexus or Navel Chakra* (from belly button to bottom of sternum)

a. Imagine a <u>yellow</u> flower opening...

b. Imagine lovingly releasing all the aka cords back to whomever they belong to and all of yours coming back to you.

c. Wonderful, now wait again a few moments while this next chakra is being cleansed

d. Know that if there are too many to release right now and you can always come back to this chakra again later,

e. Take a deep breath,

f. Imagine a clear bubble over top of this area for protection.

6. Imagine your *Heart Chakra* (between the solar plexus and your throat)

a. Imagine a <u>green</u> flower opening...

b. Imagine the aka cords being released lovingly to whomever they belong to and all of yours coming back to you.

c. Wait again a few moments while this chakra is being cleansed,

d. Take a deep breath,

e. Imagine a clear bubble over top of this area for protection.

7. Imagine your *Throat Chakra* (all your neck area)

a. Imagine a <u>blue</u> flower opening...

b. Imagine the aka being released lovingly to whomever they belong to and all of yours coming back to you.

c. Wait again while this chakra is being cleansed,

d. Take a deep breath,

e. Imagine a clear bubble over top of this area for protection.

8. Imagine your *Brow or Third eye Chakra* (your forehead area)

a. Imagine an <u>indigo</u> flower opening up...(a purple/blue color like cobalt blue)

b. Imagine all of these cords being released lovingly to whomever they belong to and all of yours coming back to you.

    c. Take a moment while this chakra is being cleansed,

    d. Take a deep breath,

    e. Imagine a clear bubble over top of this area for protection.

9. Imagine your *Crown Chakra* (top of your head, the baby soft spot)

    a. Imagine a <u>violet</u> flower opening...

    b. Imagine all of these cords being released lovingly to whomever they belong to and all of yours coming back to you.

    c. Wait for this chakra to be cleansed,

    d. Again, if there are too many to release right now and you can always come back to this chakra again later,

    e. Take a deep breath,

    f. Imagine a clear bubble over top of this area for protection.

10. Perfect, now that you have cleansed the main chakras, I want you to imagine,

    a. Beautiful crystal-clear light energy coming down from the heavens and entering your crown chakra,

    b. Let this light flow down your spinal column and up through the root chakra right up through to the crown chakra,

    c. This light flows out of the crown chakra like a water fountain and into your aura,

    d. Imagine you have an aura that is about three feet extended from you in all positions; above, behind, to the sides and below you.

    e. Bringing down from the heavens this beautiful crystal-clear light energy that continually cleanses all your chakras and flows into your aura to cleanse it as well.

    f. Now as this beautiful energy comes into your aura think positive words or affirmations,

    g. Imagine these positive words vibrating in your cleansed aura,

    h. Manifesting your drams, wishes, wants, and desires into reality.

11. Marvelous, now take a deep breath and imagine this cleansed energy being sealed into your body and aura.

12. Take another deep breath and wiggle your toes and open your eyes coming back to the moment
13. Feeling wonderfully rejuvenated and energized!

➤ B) Do some type of meditation (minimum 5 minutes) each day. It can be the candle, chakra, inner genie, negative energy clearing, relaxation, guided, or any other type of meditation you want to do today.

To help you out, I have many meditations on my Constance Santego YouTube channel.

Today, Fulfill the Goal

➤ Listen to the Negative Energy Chakra Clearing Meditation.

Bedtime

Evening Blessing
Put your hands over your Heart Center/Chakra and say this evening blessing out loud.

"Thank you to my Angels and Guides for helping me towards fulfilling my life's lessons, purpose, and journey."

Day Five

Today's Goal

- Add in Vitamins and Minerals

MORNING

1st Put your hands over your Heart Center/Chakra and say out loud the morning blessing.

2nd Do at least one round of the Eight Essential Standing Exercise

And sometime during the day go for a walk or some other kind of fitness (minimum 10 minutes).

3rd Before anything enters your mouth, bless the item(s). Follow your days plan for today's food and drink intake.

4th Do self-Reiki, (minimum 1 minute).

5th Do the 'Quick Fix' Procedure.

6th Do some type of meditation (minimum 5 minutes).

NEW Today 7th

Muscle Test if you need to take any vitamins, minerals, amino acids, or supplements today.

Muscle Test Which Ones

- If Yes, which one(s) - Go to the Vitamin page in Part Two of this book
- How many?
- When - What time of the day?

HOW TO DO MUSCLE TESTING - METHOD #2: BODY PENDULUM:
From my book, 'Secrets of a Healer – Magic of Muscle testing.'

1) Have the person stand upright.

2) Have the person lean forward from the ankles saying, "Forward is a 'yes', without falling" (the person needs to remain stiff, like a board).

3) Have the person lean backward from the ankles saying, "Backward is a 'no', without falling."

4) Have the person repeat this movement back and forward three times to program the mind.

5) Have the person practice:

a) Have him say, "My (meaning the person's name) name is _____." If he goes forward, that is correct.

b) Then practice a fake name; if he goes backward, that is correct.

c) Do a few silly, obvious questions to train him. (e.g. "My shirt color is _____.)

d) Use vitamins; have the person hold the vitamins (still in the container) and ask, "Do I need to take any today?"

If the answer is *yes*, then how many? For how many days? Add anything else you can think of.

6) Have the person then answer any other questions needed.
Remember the mind is <u>very literal</u>; it will only answer literally what you asked.

If the body sways sideways,
ask a different or more detailed question;
if it stays still/does not move, it does not know an answer.

Vitamins are great to use while learning this because the vibratory rate is so high.

¨ Now ask this question while holding the vitamins to your stomach, "Is this vitamin(s) what my body needs to have today?" Make sure your knees are relaxed and are locked neither too tightly nor loosely, just comfortably. Now allow your body to move it will either go forward or backward for the 'yes' or 'no' answer. If your body goes side to side, it means you need to ask a more specific or a better question. Try this with 5 – 10 different kinds of vitamins. When you feel confident and you can tell the difference between 'yes' and 'no', try candy or your name (if you answer incorrectly to your name, make sure you say, "in this lifetime"), or ask any other very specific single answer question you want to be answered.

Today, Fulfill the Goal

➢ Practice Muscle Testing (I have a couple of videos on my Constance Santego YouTube Channel that you can watch).

Bedtime

Evening Blessing
Put your hands over your Heart Center/Chakra and say this evening blessing out loud.

"Thank you to my Angels and Guides for helping me towards fulfilling my life's lessons, purpose, and journey."

Day Six

Today's Goal

- Muscle Test if you need to do a detoxification session

MORNING

1st Put your hands over your Heart Center/Chakra and say out loud the morning blessing.

2nd Do at least one round of the Eight Essential Standing Exercise

And sometime during the day go for a walk or some other kind of fitness (minimum 10 minutes).

3rd Before anything enters your mouth, bless the item(s). Follow your days plan for today's food and drink intake.

4th Do self-Reiki, (minimum 1 minute).

5th Do the 'Quick Fix' Procedure.

6th Do some type of meditation (minimum 5 minutes).

7th Muscle Test if you need to take any vitamins, minerals, amino acids, or supplements today.

- If Yes, which one(s) - Go to the page in Part Two of this book

NEW Today 8th Muscle Test if you need to do a specific detoxification cleanse. Refer to the 'Angelic Lifestyles, A Vibrant Lifestyle' detoxification section in that book.

Body, Mind, or Soul

- Asking, "Do I need to do a specific detoxification session for my **BODY**?"
- If Yes, which one(s)
    - Self-Reiki
    - Fasting
    - Master Cleanse
    - Homeopathy
    - Diet
    - Drink More Water
    - Respiratory Cleanse
    - Lymph & Skin Cleanse
    - Kidney & Bladder Cleanse
    - Liver & Gallbladder Cleanse
    - Contrast Shower
    - Epsom Salt Bath
    - Essential Oil Massage
    - Reflexology Session
    - Mud Wrap
    - Body Scrub or Polish
    - Colonic

- o Ear Flush
- o Teeth Cleaning
- o Cleanse my house,
  - smudge
  - crystals
  - clearing a build meditation
  - get rid of unnecessary items
    - take to garbage dump
    - donate
- o Other _____

- Asking, "Do I need to get tested?"
- If Yes, which one(s)
  - o Allergy
  - o Traditional Blood Test
  - o Blood Analysis (Holistic)
  - o Hair Analysis
  - o Saliva
  - o Urine
  - o Other _____

- Asking, "Do I need to do a specific detoxification session for my **MIND**?"
- If Yes, which one(s)
  - o Self-Reiki
  - o Self-Hypnosis or Hypnotherapy Session
  - o Take a course (online or onsite), lecture, workshop, or seminar
    - One of Constance Santego's
      - Make a list and muscle test which one
    - Other _____
  - o Read a Non-Fiction Book
    - Secrets of a Healer Series
    - Your Persona... The Mask You Wear
    - Intuitive Life

- Fairy Tales, Dreams, and Reality
- Archangel Michael's Soul Retrieval Guide
- Make your own list and muscle test which one
  - Read the Spiritual Gifts Granted by Spirit Novel Series
  - Aromatherapy
  - Bach Remedy or Flower Essence
  - Homeopathy
  - Counseling
  - Other _____

- Asking, "Do I need to do a specific detoxification session for my **SOUL**?"
- If Yes, which one(s)
  - Develop My Intuition
  - Self-Reiki
  - Pray
  - Meditate More
  - Other _____

- Asking, "Can I do the session myself?"
- If <u>Yes</u>, go ahead
- If <u>NO</u>, who do I need to go see?
  - Family Doctor
  - Naturopath
  - Health Professional
  - Natural Health or Holistic Practitioner
  - Day Spa Practitioner
  - Other _____

Today, Fulfill the Goal

> ➢ Muscle Testing if you need a specific detoxification. If you can do it yourself, go ahead. If not, then, research who to go to in your area and book an appointment.

Bedtime

Evening Blessing
Put your hands over your Heart Center/Chakra and say this evening blessing out loud.

"Thank you to my Angels and Guides for helping me towards fulfilling my life's lessons, purpose, and journey."

Day Seven

Today's Goal

- Personal Pampering Day

MORNING

1st Put your hands over your Heart Center/Chakra and say out loud the morning blessing.

2nd Do at least one round of the Eight Essential Standing Exercise

And sometime during the day go for a walk or some other kind of fitness (minimum 10 minutes).

3rd Before anything enters your mouth, bless the item(s). Follow your days plan for today's food and drink intake.

4th Do self-Reiki, (minimum 1 minute).

5th Do the 'Quick Fix' Procedure.

6th Do some type of meditation (minimum 5 minutes).

7th Muscle Test if you need to take any vitamins, minerals, amino acids, or supplements today.

8th Muscle Test if you need to do a specific detoxification session.

NEW Today **9**th Something just for you! You pick, it can be as simple as calling a friend to going on a trip. Anything that makes you happy, joyful, and creates bliss.

Muscle Test

- Paint your nails
- Dress up
- Have a relaxing bath
- Go get a hair cut
- Read a book
- Sing
- Go have a massage
- Buy something
- Go out for dinner (you can still follow your meal plan)
- Go somewhere or start to plan your next trip
    - One of Constance's Retreats
    - Other _____
- Watch your favorite show or go to a movie
- Date night
- Go out; dancing, see a performance, or sporting event
- Start writing a novel, paint, or do some other type of art
- Other _____

Today, Fulfill the Goal

> ➤ Even if all you can do today is as simple as having a bath, do that.

Bedtime

Evening Blessing
Put your hands over your Heart Center/Chakra and say this evening blessing out loud.

"Thank you to my Angels and Guides for helping me towards fulfilling my life's lessons, purpose, and journey."

Day Eight to Forty- One

Today's Goal

- Enjoy your life's journey and work towards fulfilling your life's lessons and purpose.

MORMING

1st Put your hands over your Heart Center/Chakra and say out loud the morning blessing.

2nd Do at least one round of the Eight Essential Standing Exercise

And sometime during the day go for a walk or some other kind of fitness (minimum 10 minutes).

3rd Before anything enters your mouth, bless the item(s). Follow your days plan for today's food and drink intake.

4th Do self-Reiki, (minimum 1 minute).

5th Do the 'Quick Fix' Procedure.

6th Do some type of meditation (minimum 5 minutes).

7th Muscle Test if you need to take any vitamins, minerals, amino acids, or supplements today.

8th Muscle Test if you need to do a specific detoxification session.

9th Something just for you!

NEW Today 10th

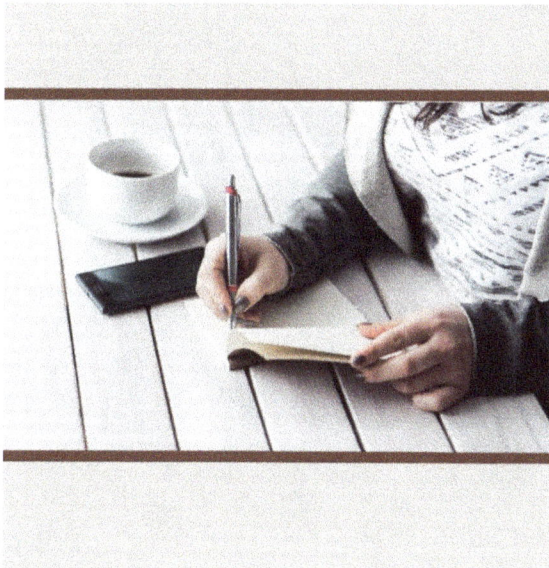

JOURNAL

If you are not already doing it, start to journal. Write in your journal what you are happy and grateful for today, make a bucket list or add to it, and if need be write out anything terrible and then rip the page out and burn it safely, while thanking your Angels and Guides for helping you to release what you do not need anymore.

FORGIVENESS RELEASE

To watch the video, go to my Constance Santego YouTube Channel.

You must clear all three aspects:
- ➢ Forgive yourself
- ➢ Forgive others
- ➢ And Allow others to forgive you

Procedure:
Say the words out loud and after each I forgive, take a deep breath & blow out into a cosmic vacuum cleaner.

Do each "I forgive "individually!

Example of 'I Forgive Myself.'

- ➢ 'I forgive myself for (1st one)' _____ ?_____ ... Take a deep breath and blow into the imaginary cosmic vacuum cleaner.
- ➢ Or you can say, 'I allow myself to forgive myself for _____ ?_____' ... Breathe

Forgive at least three things (or as many as you can think of saying). Take a breath after each I forgive.

Example of 'I Forgive Others'

- ➢ 'I forgive ____?___ for ____?___'...
  Take a breath
- ➢ 'I Allow myself to forgive ____?___ for ____?___' ... Take a breath
- ➢ 'I give myself permission to forgive ____?___ for ____?___'... Breathe

Example of 'I Allow Others To Forgive Me'
- ➤ 'I allow _____ to forgive me for _____ ?_____' ... Breathe
- ➤ I allow _____ to forgive me for _____ ?_____ ... Breathe
- ➤ I allow _____ to forgive me for _____ ?_____ ... Breathe

Stay on the topic of the issue or goal.
Use who you just forgave.
Make sure you do all the same people as before in the ' I forgive others'.

*Another great release technique is Emotional Freedom Technique. You can watch this one on my YouTube Channel also.

Today, Fulfill the Goal

- ➤ Start a Gratitude Journal.

Bedtime

Evening Blessing
Put your hands over your Heart Center/Chakra and say this evening blessing out loud.

"Thank you to my Angels and Guides for helping me towards fulfilling my life's lessons, purpose, and journey."

Day
Forty-Two

Today's Goal

- Heavenly Day

MORNING

1st Put your hands over your Heart Center/Chakra and say out loud this morning blessing.

2nd Do at least one round of the Eight Essential Standing Exercise

And sometime during the day go for a walk or some other kind of fitness (minimum 10 minutes).

NEW Today 3rd ANYTHING GOES DAY! Enjoy eating or drinking anything you want to. Before anything enters your mouth, bless the item(s).

4th Do self-Reiki, (minimum 1 minute).

5th Do the 'Quick Fix' Procedure.

6th Do some type of meditation (minimum 1 minute).

7th Muscle Test if you need to take any vitamins, minerals, amino acids, or supplements today.

8th Muscle Test if you need to do a specific detoxification session.

9th Something just for you!

10th Journal – if not doing already, start to journal.

Bedtime

Evening Blessing
Put your hands over your Heart Center/Chakra and say this evening blessing out loud.

"Thank you to my Angels and Guides for helping me towards fulfilling my life's lessons, purpose, and journey."

Now What?

Today's Goal

- Your choice, to start the 42 Day Energy Cleanse again or not. It is always your choice on how you want to live your life. I choose to live the Angelic Lifestyle's way.

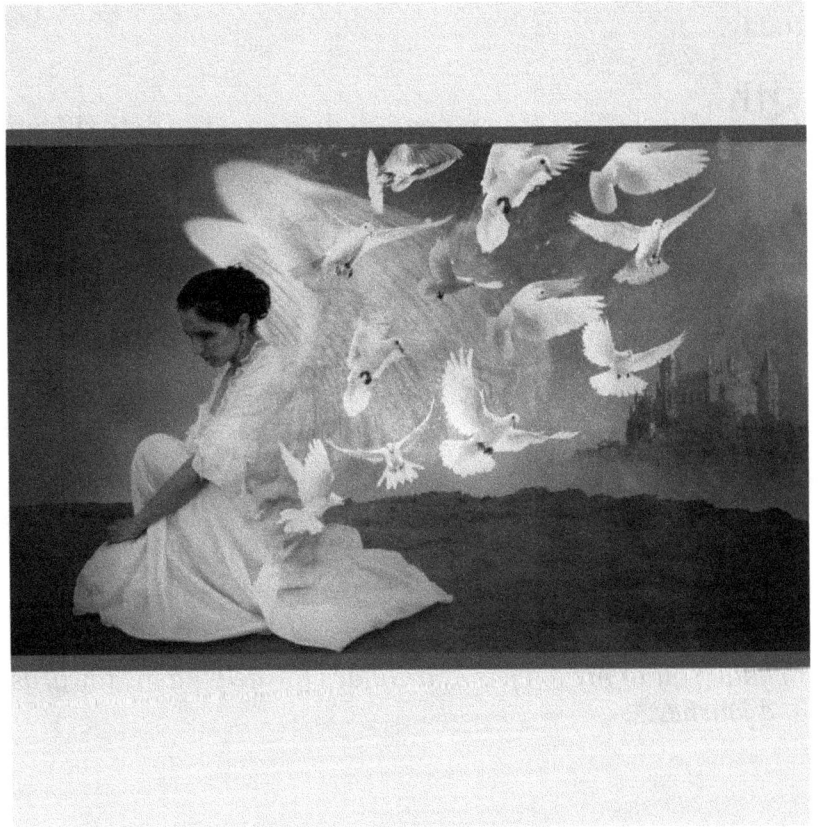

MORNING

1st Morning Blessing

"I call upon my Angels and Guides, I begin this day with gratitude, love, and abundance. I would like to thank you for helping me during the night cleanse my body, mind, and soul. I will do my best to make all that I do today empowering for my life's journey and purpose. God bless this day, the world, and everything on it. As I take my next breath, I am envisioning healing green energy and sending it out to anyone who needs it, including myself. I ask and give you permission to help guide me throughout my day... Love and Light, Namaste"

2nd Eight Essential Standing Exercises & Fitness

3rd Bless your food and drink intake

4th Self-Reiki

5th Quick Fix

6th Meditation

7th Muscle Test vitamins, minerals, amino acids, or supplements

8th Muscle Test specific detoxification session

9th Something just for you!

10th Journal (And if need be do the 'I forgive release')

Evening Blessing

Put your hands over your Heart Center/Chakra and say this evening blessing out loud.

"Thank you to my Angels and Guides for helping me towards fulfilling my life's lessons, purpose, and journey."

Part Two

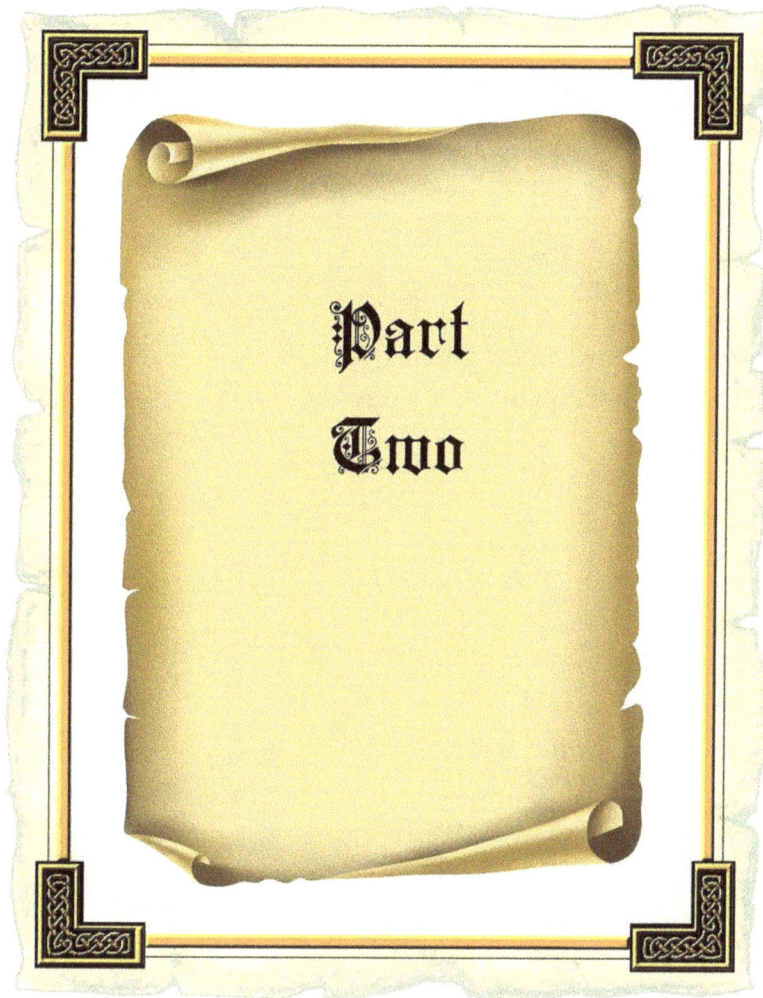

Plan and Prepare Your Meals

ANGELIC FOODS SHOPPING LIST
Purchase the items needed, for a week in advance
Do not purchase the item if you are allergic to it.

The Angelic Foods are:

SOY SAUCE

- Braggs is a healthy brand

SUGAR

(in natural form) – careful on how much you use – high in calories
- Stevia (herbal sweetener) – Powdered or liquid (also comes in flavored –chocolate raspberry or vanilla)
- Brown sugar
- Maple syrup
- Sugar cane

VINEGAR

(great for salad dressings)
- Balsamic vinegar
- Apple cider vinegar (great brand is Braggs)

PRE-MIXED SEASONINGS

- Mrs. Dash
- Cajun seasoning
- Chili seasoning
- Chinese five spice
- Greek

LIQUIDS

(up to eight glasses a day)

Water - Helps to flush toxins
- Helps to suppress your appetite
- The larger you are the more water you should drink
- Great to add some lemon to it!

Chlorophyll – green matter in plants. (Excellent in nutritional value, assist in body odor, mouth, and throat inflammation)

Tea (green tea (great antioxidant) or non-caffeinated is best)

Coffee (is a natural diuretic - need to drink more fresh water if you drink coffee)

Natural Juice (too much can be bad for your teeth; you could have half juice and add half water).

CARBOHYDRATES

(Glucose (sugar) turns into glycogen = energy; if you do not use it right away, the excess will be store in your fat cells for later use).

Simple (turns to sugar quicker)
- Whole or flaked grains only! (contains antioxidants)
  - Barley (great in soups)
  - Buckwheat
  - Corn
  - Oat
  - Quinoa
  - Rice or wild rice (brown rice takes longer for the body to turn into sugar)
  - Rye
  - Wheat (turns to sugar the quickest) A NO, NO; not ground or made into bread, pasta or noodles
- Potatoes

Complex

Vegetables – Any Type!

The first four items have less calories than it takes to eat them:
- Avocado (really a fruit)
- Celery
- Cucumber
- Lettuce
- Watercress
- Alfalfa sprouts (great nutritional value)
- Artichokes
- Arugula
- Asparagus
- Bamboo shoots
- Beans
- Bean sprouts

- Bok choy
- Broccoli (great antioxidant) – Best steamed
- Brussels sprouts – Best steamed
- Cabbage – Best steamed
- Carrots (high in sugar – but also has antioxidants)
- Cauliflower – Best steamed
- Chicory
- Chili peppers
- Dill pickles
- Eggplant
- Endive
- Green onions
- Kale – Best steamed
- Leeks
- Mushrooms
- Okra
- Olives
- Onions
- Peas
- Peppers (green, red, orange, or yellow)
- Radicchio
- Radish
- Rapini
- Snow peas
- Spaghetti squash
- Spinach (antioxidant) – Best steamed
- Swiss chard
- Tomato (really a fruit & a great antioxidant)
- Zucchini

FRUIT
ANY TYPE! (MOST FRUIT CONTAIN TRACES OF ANTIOXIDANTS)

- Apples (rich in antioxidants and two minerals called; boron – to keep bones healthy and strong & pectin – help prevent cholesterol build up)
- Apricots
- Bananas
- Berries (great antioxidants)
  - Blackberry
  - Blueberry
  - Cranberry
  - Currants
  - Figs
  - Grapefruit
  - Kiwi
  - Strawberries
  - Saskatoon berries
- Cherries
- Grapes (red - antioxidant)
- Lemons
- Limes
- Mango
- Melons
  - Honey dew
  - Cantaloupe
  - Watermelon
- Nectarines
- Oranges
- Peaches
- Pear
- Pineapple

PROTEIN

(Burns fat, but...too much can cause cholesterol problems)

- Soy milk
- Beans and Legumes
  - o Black
  - o Lima
  - o Lintels
  - o Pinto
  - o Red
  - o Red Kidney
  - o White
- Seeds (Essential fatty acids; omega 3, 6 & 9 – reduce the formation of blood clots & promotes healthy cholesterol levels, & strong bones, hair, skin and nails, & production of hormones, energy and absorption of vitamins, & regulate your metabolism).
  - - Store in the refrigerator.
    - o Flax seed (great source of protein, omega 3 & 6, lignans (have both oestrogenic and antioestrogenic activity - phytoestrogens).
    - o Pumpkin seed (also a great parasite cleanser)
    - o Sesame seed
    - o Sunflower
- Nuts (best are almonds and brazil nuts) (peanuts & cashews have more calories)
- Dairy Products
  - o Goat's milk
  - o Cow's milk (less % = Less calories)
  - o Yogurt (vanilla only, you can add you own fruit)
  - o Sour cream
  - o Cheese (including cottage & cream cheese)
  - o Butter
  - o Cream
  - o Vanilla ice cream (no more than once per week)
- Eggs

- Meat – in order of calories (try to buy lean – remove any visible fat)
  - o Fish - Any type!
    - Cod
    - Halibut
    - Sole
    - Trout
    - Tuna
    - Wild salmon (is great for improving your memory)
  - o Sea food
    - Shrimp / Prawns
    - Octopus
    - Squid (pan fried)
    - Scallops
    - Mussels
    - Oysters
    - Crab
    - Lobster
  - o Chicken (skinless)
  - o Turkey
  - o Lamb
  - o Wild meat – Moose, deer, elk, etc.
  - o Buffalo
  - o Beef
    - Steak (fat removed)
    - Extra lean ground beef
    - Any other cut
  - o Pork - Any type
    - Bacon
    - Pork chops
- Coconut milk (extremely high in calories)

FATS:

When not heated = good fats – needed for energy, production of hormones, conduction of nerve impulses, repair skin & hair, to absorb fat soluble vitamins, mental stability, bowels regulated, extra fuel if needed.

Vegetable oils

- Flax Seed oil (great for omega 3, 6 & 9 – should be refrigerated)
- Sesame Seed oil
- Extra Virgin Olive oil (refrigerated turns solid, can use as a butter, just mix with some salt first)

Vitamins, Minerals, Amino Acids & Supplements

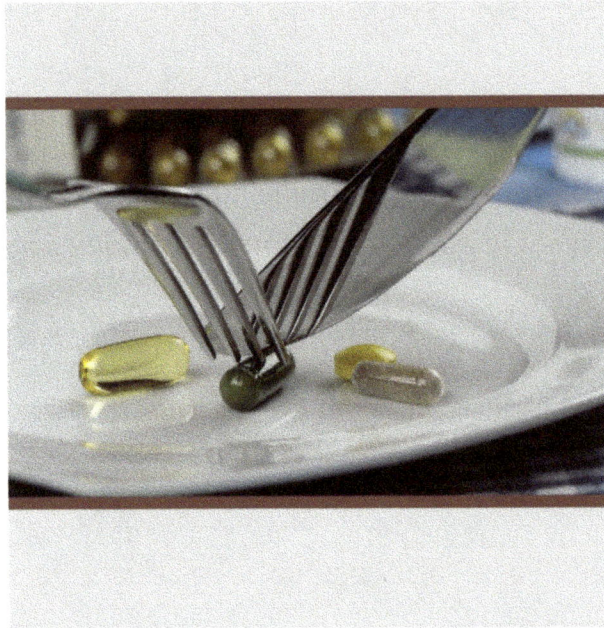

VITAMINS

Vitamins are Classified as Water-soluble or Fat Soluble

In humans there are 13 vitamins:

- 4 fat-soluble:
  - A (retinol, beta-carotene),
  - D (cholecalciferol),
  - E (d-alpha-tocopherol),
  - K (use Alfalfa, or green leafy veggies)
- 9 water-soluble
  - Vitamin C
    - Ester C,
    - bioflavonoids,
    - Hesperidin,
    - Rutin
  - 8 B vitamins
    - thiamine,
    - riboflavin,
    - niacin,
    - pantothenic acid,
    - biotin,
    - vitamin B-6 (pyridoxine),
    - vitamin B-12
    - folate
- Choline, Folic acid, Inositol, Para-aminobenzoic acid (PABA)

MINERALS

In humans there are 7 Microminerals and 13 Trace minerals (microminerals):

Microminerals

- Calcium
- Chloride
- Magnesium
- Phosphorus
- Potassium
- Sodium
- Sulfur

Trace minerals (13 Microminerals)

- Boron
- Chromium
- Copper
- Fluoride
- Iodine
- Iron
- Manganese
- Molybdenum
- Selenium
- Vanadium
- Zinc
- Iodine
- Iron

AMINO ACIDS

Amino Acids – the Building Blocks of Proteins and <u>cannot</u> be made by the body. As a result, they must come from food.

- **Aliphatic**
  - alanine,
  - glycine,
  - isoleucine,
  - leucine,
  - proline,
  - valine
- **Aromatic**
  - phenylalanine,
  - tryptophan,
  - tyrosine
- **Acidic**
  - aspartic acid,
  - glutamic acid
- **Basic**
  - arginine,
  - histidine,
  - lysine
- **Hydroxylic**
  - serine,
  - threonine
- **Sulphur**
  - cysteine,
  - methionine
- **Amidic (containing amide group)**
  - asparagine,
  - glutamine

SUPPLEMENTS

- Bee pollen
- Chondroitin sulfate
- Coenzyme A
- Coenzyme 1
- Coenzyme Q10
- Cryptoxanthin
- Flavonoids (citrus & berries)
- Free form amino acid
- Garlic
- Ginkgo biloba
- Glucosamine
- Kyo-Green
- Lecithin
- Lutein/lycopene
- Octacosanol
- Pectin
- Phosphatidyl choline
- Phosphatidyl serine
- Protein powder
- Pycnogenol or grape seed extract
- Quercetin
- RNA-DNA
- Siberian ginseng
- Silicon
- Soy isoflavones (genistein)
- Spirulina
- Superoxide dismutase (SOD)
- Wheat germ
- Zeaxanthin

Make your Angelic Foods Shopping List

Carbohydrates

_____ _____ _____ _____
_____ _____ _____ _____
_____ _____ _____ _____

Proteins

_____ _____ _____ _____
_____ _____ _____ _____

Fats

_____ _____ _____ _____

Seasonings

_____ _____ _____ _____
_____ _____ _____ _____

Liquids

_____ _____ _____ _____
_____ _____ _____ _____

Vitamins, Minerals, Amino Acids, or Supplements

_____ _____ _____ _____
_____ _____ _____ _____

Measurements & Quick Conversion

Cooking Abbreviation(s)	Unit of Measurement
C, c	cup
g	gram
kg	kilogram
L, l	liter
lb	pound
mL, ml	milliliter
oz	oz
pt	pint
q, qt, fl qt	quart
g, gal	gallon
t, tsp	tsp
T, TB, Tbl, Tbsp	Tablespoon

Volume (liquid)					
			32 qt		1 bushel
256 Tbsp	16 C	3.8 L	4 qt	1 g	8 pt
128 Tbsp	8 C	1.9 L	2 qt	½ g	4 pt
64 Tbsp	4 C	946 ml	1 qt	32 fl oz	2 pt
32 Tbsp	2 C	473 ml		16 fl oz	1 pt
16 Tbsp	1 C	137 ml	½ pt	8 fl oz	½ pt
12 Tbsp	¾ C	177 ml		6 fl oz	
	2/3 C	158 ml			
8 Tbsp	½ C	118 ml	¼ pt	4 fl oz	1 stick of butter
5 Tbsp & 1 tsp	1/3 C	79 ml		2.7 fl oz	
4 Tbsp	¼ C	59 ml		2 fl oz	
				1 ½ fl oz	1 jigger
2 Tbsp	1/8 C	30 ml		1 fl oz	
1 Tbsp	1/16 C	15 ml	3 tsp	.5 fl oz	180 drops
1 tsp		5 ml	5 g	.176 oz	60 drops
¾ tsp		3.7 ml			45 drops
½ tsp		2.5 ml			30 drops
¼ tsp		1.2 ml			15 drops
1/8 tsp		.6 ml		Dash or pinch	

Volume (mass & weight)		
½ oz	14 grams	
1 oz	28 grams	
3 oz	85 grams	
3.53 oz	100 grams	
4 oz	113 grams	
8 oz	227 grams	
12 oz	340 grams	
16 oz	454 grams	1 pound

Safe Cooking Temperatures

Cook foods to the recommended safe minimum internal temperature listed below.

Beef & Veal
Ground	160 ºF
Steak and roasts medium	160 ºF
Steak and roasts medium rare	145 ºF

Chicken & Turkey
Breasts	165 ºF
Ground, stuffing, and casserole	165 ºF
Whole bird, legs, thighs, and wings	
	165 ºF

Eggs
Any type	160 ºF

Fish & Shellfish
Any type	145 ºF

Lamb
Ground	160 ºF
Steak and roasts medium	160 ºF
Steak and roasts medium rare	145 ºF

Leftovers
Any type	165 ºF

Pork
Chops, fresh (raw) ham ground, ribs and roasts	160 ºF
Fully cooked ham (to reheat)	140 ºF

One of the Secrets to Cooking is...
Spices and Herbs

SPICES AND HERBS

Herbs are usually from the leaves, such as Basil, Thyme or Chives, and spices are usually from the root or seeds, such as Black Pepper, Salt or Cinnamon.

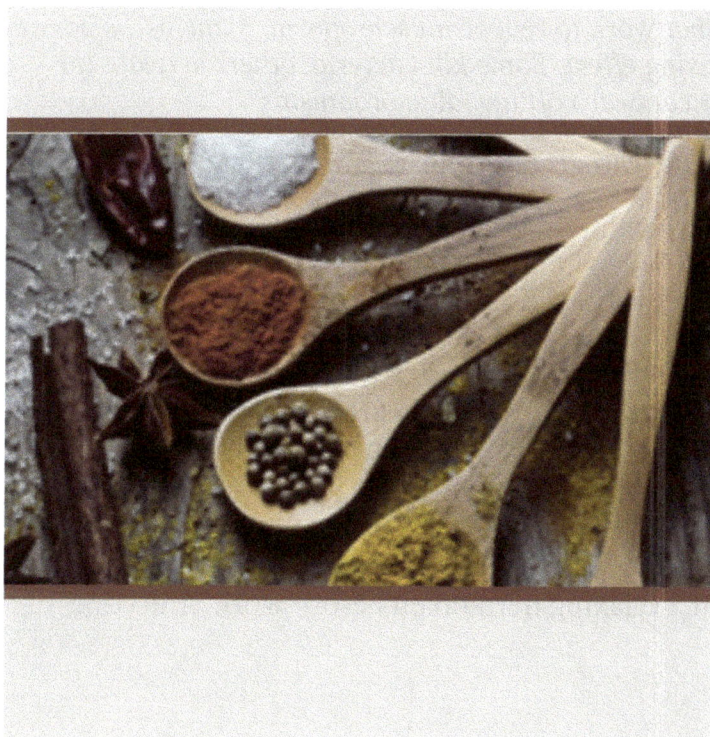

Botany is the science of plants, and horticulture is the art or science of growing the plants.

Herbs are great to add to the taste of your food, but did you know they can also assist by:
It is important to visit your local **Naturopath, Herbalist, or Doctor** for further assistance when taking herbs. Although herbs are natural, they can be very powerful and should be used with respect.

1. Fighting infection
2. Clearing congestion
3. Soothing inflammation
4. Calming Spasm
5. Opening Airways

How Herbs Work

The cells of a plant take carbon dioxide, water, and sunlight (photosynthesis) and turn it into useful nutrients. Oxygen is a byproduct of this process. Many herbs are rich in compounds that are beneficial and have profound healing effects on tissue and organs.

Master Herbalist, Earl Mindell quotes:

> *"There are herbs that target specific organs systems and there are herbs that are used as general tonics to promote overall heath. There are herbs that soothe pain and inflammation, and still other herbs that work to reduce muscle spasm. Some herbs have a stimulating effect; others have a relaxing effect. Some kill bacteria: others activate the body's own immune system so that it can ward off invading organisms".*

Generally, medicinal herbs fall into two basic categories: tonic & stimulating

> Tonics help cells, tissues, & organs to maintain tone, or balance, throughout the body.
> Stimulating herbs have much stronger actions & are used to treat particular ailments.

Just like medicine there are many cautions of using herbs:

- Herbs to Avoid for High Blood Pressure: Avoid strong heart stimulants & herbs that constrict blood vessels, except in small quantities. (Golden Seal, Ginseng, Licorice) Cayenne & Garlic are permitted.
- If taken too often or for too long
- Mixed improperly, needs to be balanced with all systems of the body
- Stimulating herb taken at night and a relaxing herb taken before work or driving
- Taken with modern medicine
- Taken with alcohol or drugs
- Taken on an empty stomach
- Wrong dosage for the size of person

Growing Your Own Herbs

How and when to use herbs

Gathering should be undertaken at the right time, at the right place & in the right manner. Fresh herbs can be picked in early spring (end of February), into November. Some can even be found during the winter under the snow if you know where to look.

The optimum times to gather herbs are as follows:

Leaves -   Spring/Summer (Before & during the time of flowering)

Blossoms -   Summer (Pick flowers at the beginning of flowering)

Roots -   Fall/Spring (Dig in early spring or autumn)

Fruits -   Gather at the time of ripening.

Pick only healthy, clean plants free from pests and contaminants. Gather herbs on sunny days in dry conditions, after the dew has evaporated. *Be considerate of Nature.* Do not pull plants out by their roots. Do not girdle a tree. Do not crush flowers and leaves while gathering. Do not use plastic bags and containers. The herbs will begin to sweat and later turn black during drying. Do not cut more than 20% of the plant. It will die if too much is taken.

Do not wash herbs before drying. Bundle and hang to dry in a well-ventilated area away from sunlight. Herbs must be fully dried before putting into storage jars. Dark colored glass jars are recommended. Avoid plastic and metal containers.

With time herbs lose their healing powers so it is recommended to keep a supply for one winter only. Every year blesses us with a new harvest of herbs. *Most importantly remember to give thanks.*

Dried herbs use half the number of fresh herbs. Dried herbs are shrunken in size but still very powerful.

Cooking with Herbs

- Cayenne releases endorphins for pain control.
- Cinnamon stimulates the circulation & is taken as a warming herb. It can be combined with ginger to relieve aching muscles and cold symptoms. It is also a classic remedy for digestive problems.
- Coriander, cumin, and ginger are used in bean dishes to combat flatulence.
- Foods will generally digest better with the addition of cinnamon, cloves, coriander, ginger, nutmeg, and cardamom as the have expansive, drying, and warming qualities. These include yams, sweet potatoes, winter squash, as well as sweet and mucous forming foods.
- Garlic and ginger are good cold remedies.
- Garlic is effective for treating all lung ailments, hi and low blood pressure, infections, nervous disorders, headaches, and parasites.
- Ginger is used to help breakdown meat, beans, and other high protein foods.
- In Chinese Medicine cloves have been used to treat indigestion, diarrhea, hernia, ringworm, and athlete's foot and other fungal infections.
- In Chinese Medicine nutmeg is used for intestinal problems and diarrhea. Large doses are poisonous and could cause miscarriage.
- In Indian Ayurvedic medicine cloves are used to treat respiratory and digestive problems.
- Indian Ayurvedic practitioners recommend drinking equal amounts of cumin, coriander, and fennel in a tea to clear up acne. 1 tsp of the combined herbs steeped for 10 minutes in 1 cup of water.
- In Egypt cumin is a popular spice and medicinal herb used for illnesses of the digestive tract, to treat coughs and chest colds, and to relieve pain, particularly for toothache.
- In Indian Ayurvedic medicine turmeric is considered a natural antibiotic that can also strengthen digestion and improve intestinal flora. Large amounts of turmeric can upset the stomach.
- Plants from the mint family are the richest sources of antioxidants. These include oregano, rosemary, thyme, sage, peppermint, and spearmint.
- Parsley root can be used to dissolve kidney and gall bladder stones.

- Steep several springs of rosemary in boiled water and drink daily to stay mentally sharp. This can also be added to the bath as the antioxidants can be absorbed by the skin.
- Seven corns of black pepper ground with honey taken 3 to 4 times per day is a good remedy for mucous and sore throats.

Shelf Life of Herbs

- Dried herbs should be as fresh as possible; up to one year, and then throw away.
- Decoctions and Teas should be used up in a couple of days.
- Tinctures two years.
- Unopened containers of tablets and capsules are good up to two years - opened, one year

Basic Herbal First Aid Kit

- Arnica gel ointment and tincture for sprains, bruises, or muscle strain.
- Calendula cream is used as an all-purpose skin healer
- Echinacea - tincture or capsules for colds and the flu
- Ginger capsules or tea for motion sickness, upset stomach and nausea
- Lavender counteracts stress and aids sleep
- Peppermint oil for headaches. Also aids in staying awake
- Rescue Remedy emotional trauma care
- Tea Tree Oil antibiotic, antiseptic, and antiviral

IF YOU BURN YOURSELF

- Aloe Vera gel
- Apply 5 - 10 drops of Lavender Essential Oil *Lavandula angustafolia* neat (pure) onto the burned area, and then use a zip lock bag full of ice to bring down the temperature. Repeat as needed.

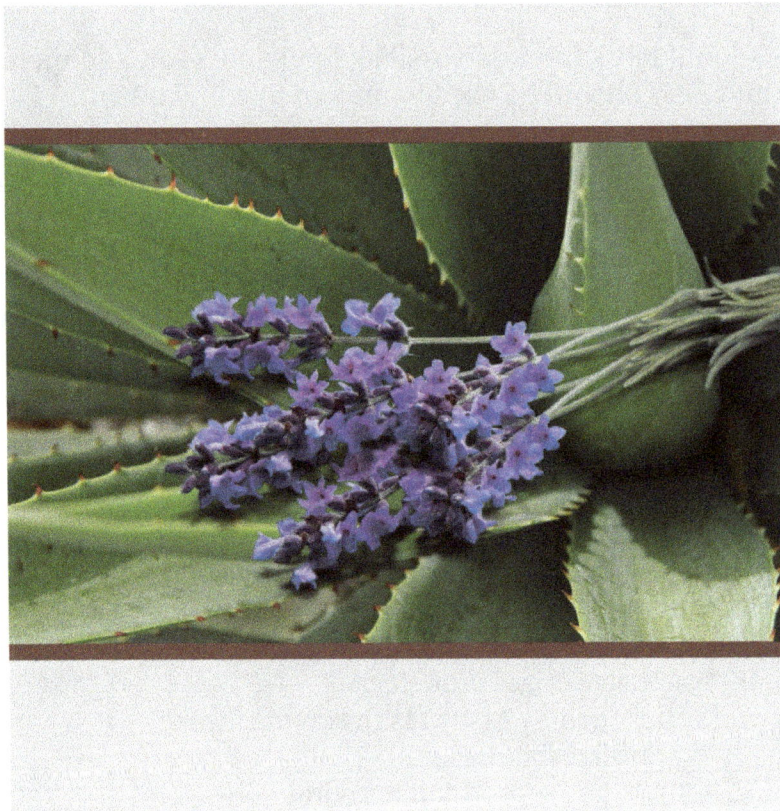

Most Common Herbs and Spices
used in Cooking

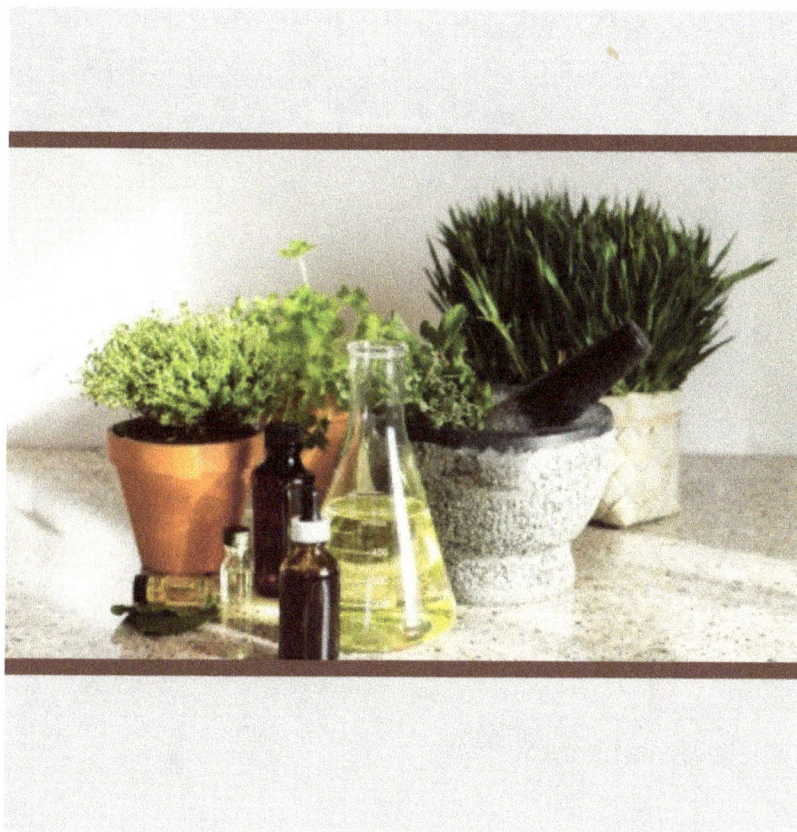

Allspice   Whole or ground
- The whole berries are used in pickling, casseroles, and soups.
- Ground is used in baking

Anise seed   Whole or ground
- It has a licorice flavour
- Used in baking and in ethnic foods

Basil   Fresh or dried
- Used in fish, veal, pork and lamb
- Salads and Tomato based dishes

Bay Leaf   Fresh or dried ("bouquet garni"- for flavour only – removed before serving)
- Spaghetti sauce
- Stews, meats dishes and pickling

Borage   Fresh or dried
- Tomato or Mustard sauces
- Salads and vegetables

Caraway   Seeds
- Meat dishes, potatoes, cabbage, soups, and sauces.

Cardamom   Whole or ground
- Pickling and curried dishes
- Ground in baking

Cayenne   Dried or powder
- Chilli, fish, beef, and pork

Chilies   Fresh or powder
- Mexican cooking

Chives   Copped fresh or dried
- Tastes a bit like onions
- Soups, salads, sauces, and egg
- As a garnish

Cinnamon   Ground or stick
- Sweet dishes
- Milk puddings, stewed fruit

Cloves   Whole or ground
- Meat, vegetable, soups, sauces, stewed fruit
- Remove whole clove from dish before eating!

Coriander   Powder or seeds
- Meat dishes

Curry   Powder
- Indian cooking
- Veal, beef, lamb, pork, and chicken casseroles
- Shrimp and vegetable dishes

Dill   Fresh or dried
- Fish, beef, and lamb
- Vegetables, salads
- Eggs

Fennel   Fresh or dried
- Fish, salads, mushrooms
- It has a licorice flavour

Garlic   Powder, roots –finely chopped or crushed
- Fish, meat and poultry dishes
- Salads, sauces, cheese, salad dressings and mayonnaise

Ginger   Powder, Roots –finely chopped or crushed
- Sugar, syrup
- Tea and baking

Horseradish roots grated or powder
- Cream as a sauce
- Beef, ham

Juniper   Berries
- Meat and game

Marjoram   Leaves fresh or dried (may cause emotional numbness)
- Pork, poultry, and game stew
- Soups or sauces

Mint   Fresh or dried
- Stuffing, peas, new potatoes
- salads

Mustard   Seeds, ground, or powder
- pickling,
- meat, cheese, poultry dishes, sauces, and marinades

Nutmeg   Whole, ground, or powder
- Potato, spinach, cauliflower
- Soups, sauces and cheese and baking

Oregano   fresh, dried or powder
- Italian dishes
- Vegetable, meat, tomato sauces

Paprika   Ground or powder
- Fish, meat
- Vegetable, soups, sauces, and salad dressings

Parsley   Fresh or dried
- Savoury dishes (salt or spicy)
- garnish

Pepper   Whole, ground, or powder
- Savoury dishes (salt or spicy)
- Black for dark foods
- White for pale coloured foods (like fish or poultry)

Rosemary   Fresh or dried
- Pork, lamb, veal, and chicken
- Garnish

Saffron   Powder
- Fish, chicken
- Rice
- Curries

Sage   Fresh or dried
- Pork, Goose, duck
- Savoury dishes (salt or spicy)
- Soups

Savory   Fresh or Dried
- Fish, poultry, meat
- Vegetable

Tarragon   Fresh or dried
- Vinegar
- Egg, fish, and poultry
- Sauces, savory butters
- Salads and vegetables

Thyme   Fresh or dried
- Fish, meat, and poultry
- Stuffing, sauces, and soups

SPICES & HERBS MAKE FOOD EXCITING!

Change up your cooking by adding a new taste. The same potato can be cooked many ways; shape, size, and what spices or herbs you add to it.
Same food different experience!

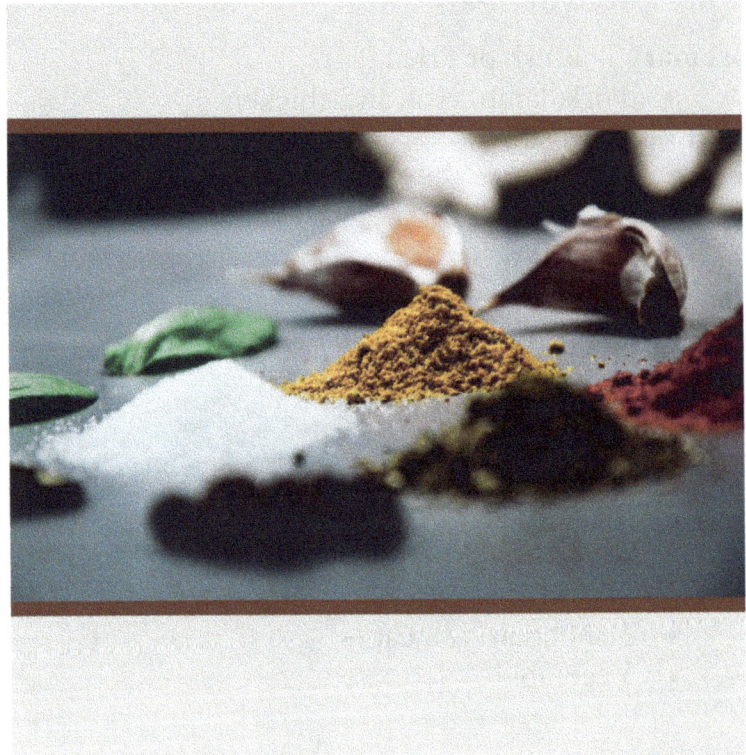

SPICES

(Fresh, dried, or powdered)
- Celery seed
- Cinnamon
- Cloves
- Cocoa
- Coriander seed
- Curry powder
- Garlic (great antioxidants)
- Ginger (fresh - makes a great tea)
- Horse radish
- Mustard
- Onion
- Pepper
  - Black
  - Cayenne
  - Red
- Poppy seeds
- Salt (sea salt is best)
- Turmeric
- Vanilla

SEASONINGS

Herbs – Any type!

- Basil
- Bay Leaf (cannot eat – just to add flavor)
- Chives
- Cilantro
- Dill
- Fennel
- Marjoram *(careful – can nullify emotions and sex drive)*
- Mint
- Oregano
- Parsley
- Rosemary
- Sage
- Savory
- Tarragon
- Thyme

INTERESTING FACTS

- Alfalfa (must be used in fresh form to provide all nutrients)
- Astragalus (should not be taken if fever is present)
- Cayenne pepper (avoid contact with broken skin, eyes and mucous membranes)
- Echinacea (Avoid or use moderately - if pregnant, acute inflammation or pain in kidneys)
- Goldenseal herb (should not be used if pregnant, or for prolonged periods)
- Licorice root (there are many cautions with this herb, use under the supervision of the qualified herbalist or naturopath)
- Lemongrass (no known cautions)
- Milk Thistle (no known cautions)
- Mullein leaf (no known cautions)
- Nettle (no known cautions)
- Peppermint leaf (do not ingest pure essential oil, should not be used by nursing mothers)
- Rosehips (good source of Vitamin C)
- Sage leaf (interferes with iron absorption, do not take if pregnant or a history of seizure disorders)
- Stevia leaf (no known cautions)

Meal Plan Chart

Write down what you are eating (If you are eating more often, just write in the times).

Meals

Date:_____	Time of day	Food Eaten	Liquid
Breakfast	_____	_____	_____
Lunch	_____	_____	_____
Dinner	_____	_____	_____
Snack	_____	_____	_____

Date:_____	Time	Food Eaten	Liquid
Breakfast	_____	_____	_____
Lunch	_____	_____	_____
Dinner	_____	_____	_____
Snack	_____	_____	_____

Date:_____	Time	Food Eaten	Liquid
Breakfast	_____	_____	_____
Lunch	_____	_____	_____
Dinner	_____	_____	_____
Snack	_____	_____	_____

Date:_____	Time	Food Eaten	Liquid
Breakfast	_____	_____	_____
Lunch	_____	_____	_____
Dinner	_____	_____	_____
Snack	_____	_____	_____

Date:_____	Time	Food Eaten	Liquid
Breakfast	_____	_____	_____
Lunch	_____	_____	_____
Dinner	_____	_____	_____
Snack	_____	_____	_____

Date:_____	Time	Food Eaten	Liquid
Breakfast	_____	_____	_____
Lunch	_____	_____	_____
Dinner	_____	_____	_____
Snack	_____	_____	_____

Date:_____	Time	Food Eaten	Liquid
Breakfast	_____	_____	_____
Lunch	_____	_____	_____
Dinner	_____	_____	_____
Snack	_____	_____	_____

Part Three

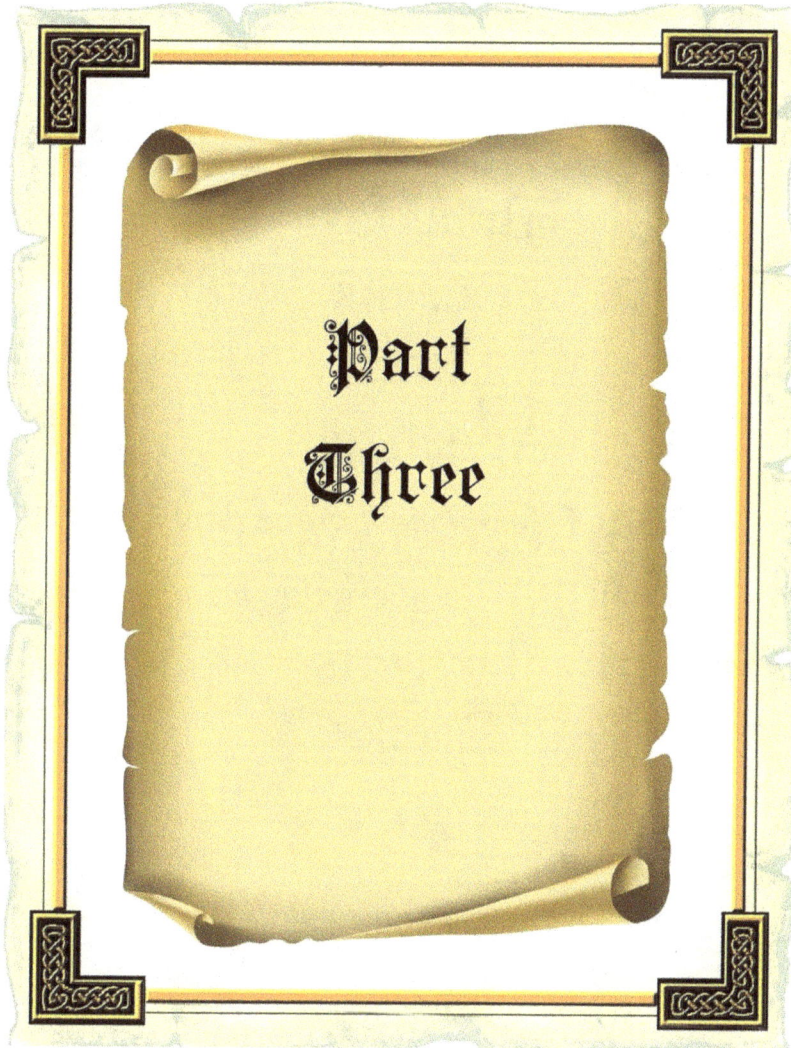

Great Recipe Ideas

Breakfast
Snacks
Lunch
Appetizers
Dinner *(main meal of the day)* or
Supper *(light evening meal)*
Desserts
Drinks

Breakfast

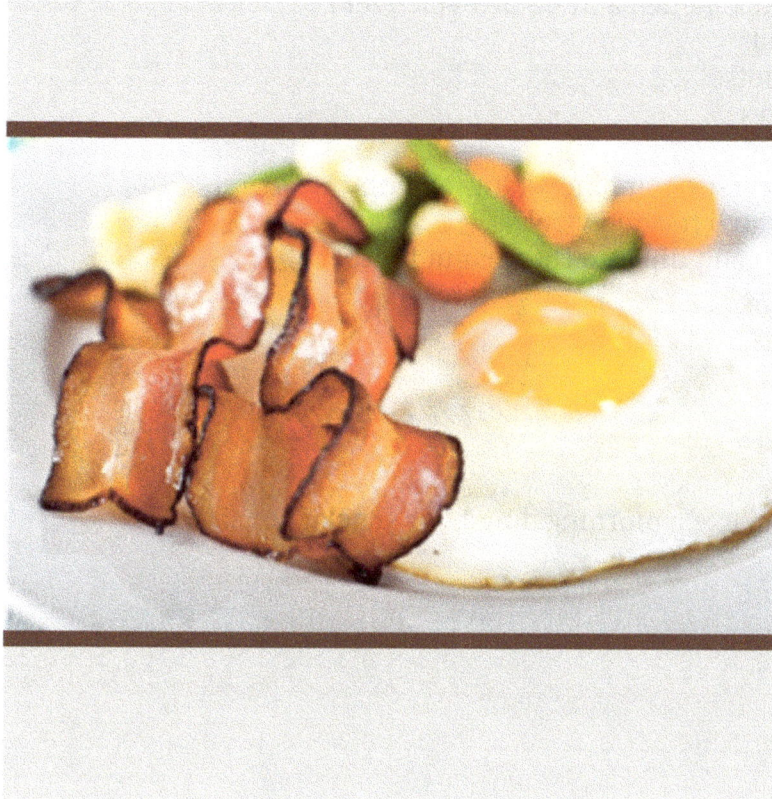

Banana and Peanut Butter

You choose; one or all, 2 cups nuts to ½ cup olive oil
½ cup peanuts (shelled and no brown cover)
½ cup almonds
½ cup hazelnuts
½ cup cashews
½ cup olive oil
In a food processor combine all ingredients and grind.
Keep refrigerated for two weeks.
Cut up banana and dip into the peanut butter.

Fruit Ideas:

Any kind, or make a morning, lunch, or snack fruit salad.

Cauliflower Bread

Line a 9"-x-5" loaf pan with parchment paper.

3 cups cauliflower, riced (chop in blender)
6 large eggs, separated
1 ¼ cups almond flour
1 tbsp baking powder
1 tsp salt
6 tbsp melted butter

Optional
5 cloves garlic, minced
1 tbsp freshly chopped thyme
1 tbsp freshly chopped parsley
Freshly grated Parmesan or cheddar, for serving

Boil cauliflower until soft and tender. Let cool. When cool enough to handle, transfer cauliflower to a clean kitchen towel and squeeze out as much moisture as possible. Put back into a bowl.

In a medium bowl, beat egg whites until stiff peaks form. Set aside.

In a large bowl, whisk together almond flour, baking powder, salt, egg yolks, melted butter, *(garlic - if using),* and about a quarter of the whipped egg whites. Beat until well combined, then stir into the cauliflower.

Fold in the remaining egg whites and mix until fluffy.

(if using, fold in the thyme and most of the parsley (save some for topping).

Transfer batter to prepared pan *(and sprinkle with remaining herbs).*

Bake at 350°until the top is golden, about 45 to 50 minutes.

Let cool completely before slicing. Sprinkle slices with Parmesan and more parsley before serving.

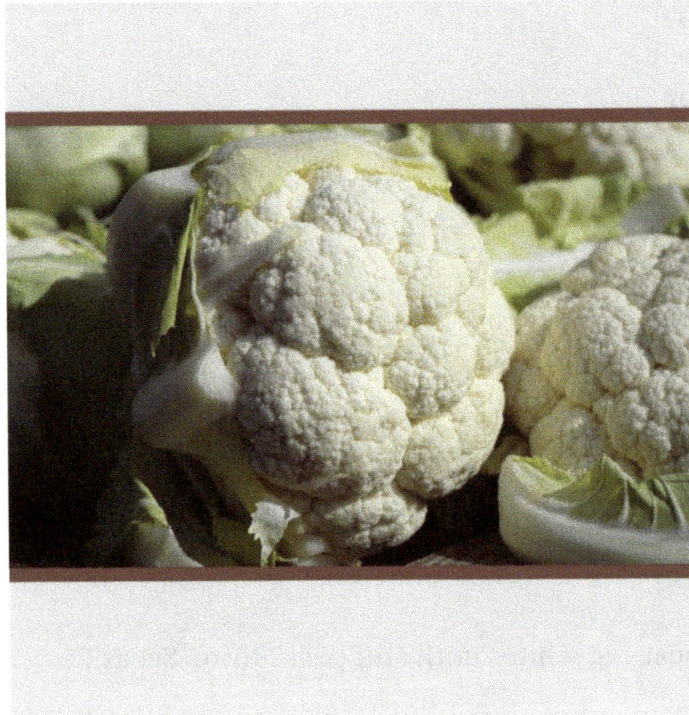

Crunchy Granola

Oven 250º
30 -50 minutes

5 cups Oats flaked, or rye, or wheat, or combination
1 cup sesame seeds
1 cup sunflower seeds
1 cup pumpkin seeds
1 cup wheat germ
1 cup flax
1 cup bran
2 Tbsp cinnamon
1 cup of chopped nuts (optional)
      - pecans, almonds and or walnuts
1 cup of coconut
1 cup vegetable oil
1 cup honey

1 cup of each: Dried cranberries, dates raisins, peaches, banana, apple, blueberries, cherries, apricots, or a combination.

In a large bowl mix dry ingredient together. In a pot on the stove heat the oil and honey together 5-8 minutes. Pour the oil and honey into the dry mixture and stir. On two cookie sheets divide mixture evenly and spread out. The thinner it is spread the faster it will brown (watch often so it does not burn). Place into oven for 30 -50 minutes. Remove from oven and let cool.
Once cooled add dried fruit and stir.

To eat take ½ to 1 cup of granola mix and pour milk over and eat as a cereal or instead of milk try adding fresh or thawed fruit and vanilla or plain yogurt.

Eggs

Fried

In medium saucepan, melt 1 tsp of butter. Crack eggs (with no shells) into pan, careful not to break the yoke. On medium / low heat add salt and pepper to taste. Place lid over pan and let sit 1 -3 minutes check to see if runniness is gone.

Hardboiled

In medium pot place whole eggs into water, water should cover the eggs. Place on burner and boil for ten minutes. Remove from heat and drain water, replace by filling the pot with cold water and let eggs sit for five to ten minutes. Remove from water and crack and peel shell off. Wash quickly under water, paper towel dry and set on plate. Sprinkle with salt and pepper to taste and eat.

Omelette

In medium saucepan, melt 1 tsp of butter. Crack eggs (with no shells) into bowl and beat. On medium / low heat add eggs, salt and pepper to taste and stir. This is when you add the extra ingredients; onion, green peppers, green onion, mushrooms, chopped tomato, cheese anything you like. Optional; Ham, bacon, crab.
Cook all until runniness is gone

Over easy

In medium saucepan, melt 1 tsp of butter. Crack eggs (with no shells) into pan, careful not to break the yoke. On medium / low heat add salt and pepper to taste. Let sit 2 -3 minutes, until runniness is almost all gone. Using a flipper; flip the egg onto the other side and let sit 1 minute.

Poached

- Use a pan or a pot that is at least 3-inches deep so there is enough water to cover the eggs, and they do not stick to the bottom of the pan.
- You will want to bring the water to a temperature of about 160 to 180°F (71-82°C). If the water is too cool, the egg will separate apart before it cooks; if your water is too hot, you will end up with tough whites and an over-cooked yolk. To obtain the correct temperature, spin the boiling water with a spoon to cool down the water before you drop in the egg.

Hints:

If you do not mind the taste of a little white vinegar with your poached eggs, try adding a couple teaspoons of vinegar to the water. Vinegar helps the egg to hold its shape by causing the outer layer of the egg white to congeal faster.

Do not add salt, which would do the opposite and loosen the whites.

- Slip eggs carefully into slowly or gently simmering water by lowering each egg ½ -inch below the surface of the water.
- Let the eggs flow out. Do not put too many eggs in the pot at one time.
- With a spoon, gently nudge the egg whites closer to their yolks.
- Immediately cover with a lid and turn off the heat. Do not disturb the egg/eggs once you have put it in the water!
- Set a timer for exactly 3 minutes for medium-firm yolks. Adjust the time up or down for runnier or firmer yolks. Cook 3 to 5 minutes, depending on firmness desired. You can test for softness/firmness by lifting an egg on a spoon and gently pressing a finger on the yolk.
- Remove from water with slotted spoon but hold it over the skillet briefly to let any water clinging to the egg drain off. Remove each egg in succession after they have each cooked for the doneness you want.

Optional: Put the finished poached eggs in a bowl of cold water. This stops the cooking.

Scrambled Eggs

In medium saucepan, melt 1 tsp of butter. Crack eggs (with no shells) into bowl and beat. On medium / low heat add eggs, salt and pepper to taste and stir until runniness is gone (some people like soft scrambled and some people like dry scrambled).

Veggie & Cheese Frittata

Baked frittata is like an omelette or quiche. It is an egg-based dish that may be flavoured with herbs and additional ingredients such as meats, cheeses, and vegetables (Great for breakfast, brunch, lunch, or supper).

350°
45 minutes 6 servings

¼ cup milk
6 eggs, slightly beaten
½ cup (1 medium) chopped onion
¼ tsp salt
¼ tsp pepper
½ tsp dried basil leaves
3 Tbsp butter
½ tsp finely chopped fresh garlic

Handful of spinach (fifteen pieces)
1 cup (1 medium) diagonally sliced ¼ inch zucchini
1 medium ripe tomato, cut into 6 slices
3 large sliced mushrooms
¼ cup (1 oz) shredded Mozzarella cheese
¼ cup (1 oz) shredded Cheddar cheese
2 Tbsp freshly grated Parmesan cheese

Heat oven. In medium bowl stir together milk, eggs, onion, salt, and pepper. In ovenproof 10-inch skillet melt butter over medium heat; stir in garlic. Pour egg mixture into skillet. Bake for 10 minutes or until egg is partially set. Remove from oven. Arrange spinach and zucchini on top of egg mixture; place tomato slices on top of zucchini; add sliced mushrooms on top of tomatoes. Top with green onions. Sprinkle with the three cheeses. Continue baking for 12 -15 minutes or until eggs are set in center and cheese is melted. Remove from oven (Careful handle is hot!).

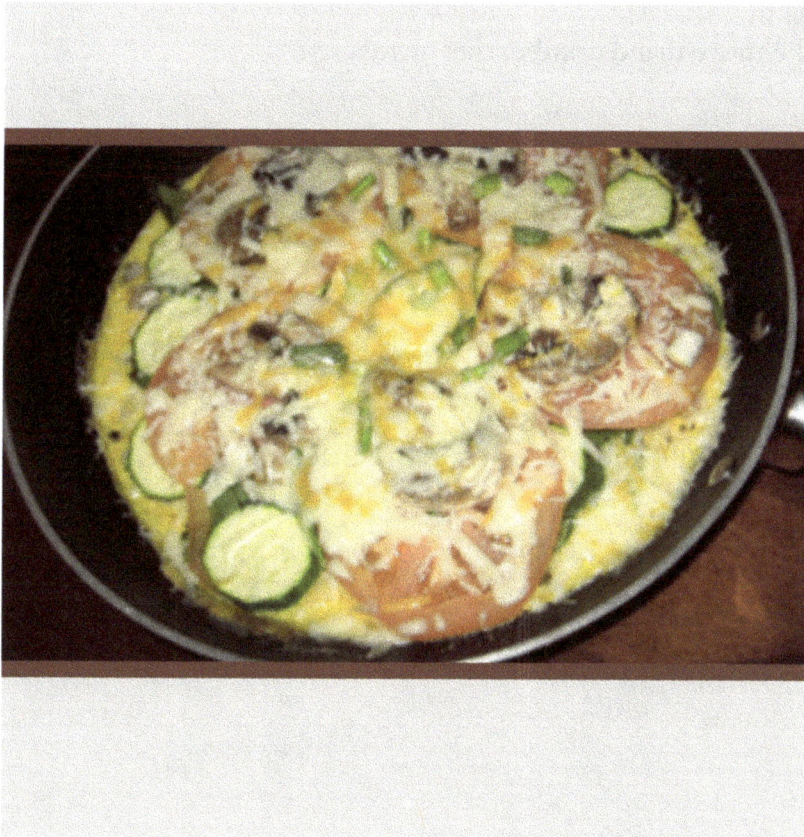

Flax Plus Cereal

SERVES ONE
1 ½ cups
1 cup Milk
¼ cup cranberries and or raisins

In bowl pour the cereal in.
Add milk and if you like more dried cranberries or raisins.

Two Scoops of Raisin Bran

SERVES ONE
1 ½ cups
1 cup Milk
¼ cup Raisins

In bowl pour cereal in. Add milk and if you like more dried raisins.

Shredded Wheat

SERVES ONE
2 of the Regular
1 cup Milk
Maximum 3 Tbsp Brown sugar
Turn water tap to hot and let heat up. In bowl place two of the Shredded Wheat. Pour the hot tap water over and saturate the Shredded Wheat and drain quickly.   Pour milk over. Sprinkle brown sugar over top.

Weetabix

Weetabix is a whole-grain wheat breakfast cereal

SERVES ONE
2 of the Weetabix
1 cup Milk
Maximum 3 Tbsp Brown sugar
In bowl place two of the Weetabix. Pour milk over. Sprinkle brown sugar over top.

Oatmeal

SERVES ONE
1/3 cup Large flake oats from Robin Hood
Pinch of salt
1 cup water
½ tsp Butter
Maximum 3 Tbsp Brown sugar
½ tsp cinnamon
Dash of milk

In large microwave-safe bowl, gradually stir oats into cold, salted water. Heat uncovered on high power for 1 ½ to 2 minutes, stir after 1 minute. Stir again; let stand 1 minute. Add butter, brown sugar, cinnamon, and milk. Stir.

Porridge

SERVES ONE
1/3 cup Red River from Smuckers/Robin Hood
Pinch of salt
1 cup water
½ tsp Butter
Maximum 3 Tbsp Brown sugar
½ tsp cinnamon
Dash of milk

In large microwave-safe bowl, gradually stir Red River into cold, salted water. Heat uncovered on high power for 1 ½ to 2 minutes, stir after 1 minute. Stir again; let stand 1 minute. Add butter, brown sugar, cinnamon, and milk. Stir.

Pancakes

1 cup Almond Flour
¼ cup water or milk
2 large eggs
1 Tbsp maple syrup or vanilla extract
¼ tsp cinnamon
¼ tsp salt
¼ tsp baking soda
1 tsp olive oil or butter
Optional, 1 Tbsp chocolate chips, diced apple, or blueberries

Mix almond flour, water, eggs, maple syrup, cinnamon, salt, and baking soda together in a bowl until batter is smooth.

Heat oil in a skillet over medium heat; drop large spoonsful of batter onto the griddle and cook until bubbles form and the edges are dry, 3 to 5 minutes.
Flip, and cook the other side, 3 to 5 minutes.

Repeat with remaining batter.
Top with your favorite toppings and serve.

Potatoes for Breakfast

Hash Browns

Dice potato into small pieces
Melt butter in a fry pan on the stove
Add potatoes stir & flip, cut until tender
Add spices & onions if desired

Re-Fried Smashed Potatoes

Maybe use leftovers from last night <u>or</u> Boil potatoes until tender
Drain water
Add ½ cup of milk and 1 tsp butter
Smash till smooth and soft
Melt butter in a fry pan on the stove
Add smashed potatoes
Flip as needed, should brown

Silver Dollars

Peel, or not, the potato
Slice into thin pieces. Should look like the size of silver dollars or loonies
Melt butter in a fry pan on the stove
Add potatoes stir & flip, cut until tender
Add spices & onions if desired

Smoothie

– SEE DRINKS

Traditional Breakfast

Cooked Meat (Bacon, ham, steak)
Eggs (any style)
Fried diced potatoes, optional butter
Fresh or cooked sliced tomatoes
Cook with any combination of your favourite herbs, spices, and cheese

Yogurt Breakfast or Snack

1 cup of plain or fruit flavoured yogurt
¼ cup sliced or diced fruit (any type)
3 Tbsp Flax Plus from Nature's Path or Crunchy Granola
Mix together

Snacks

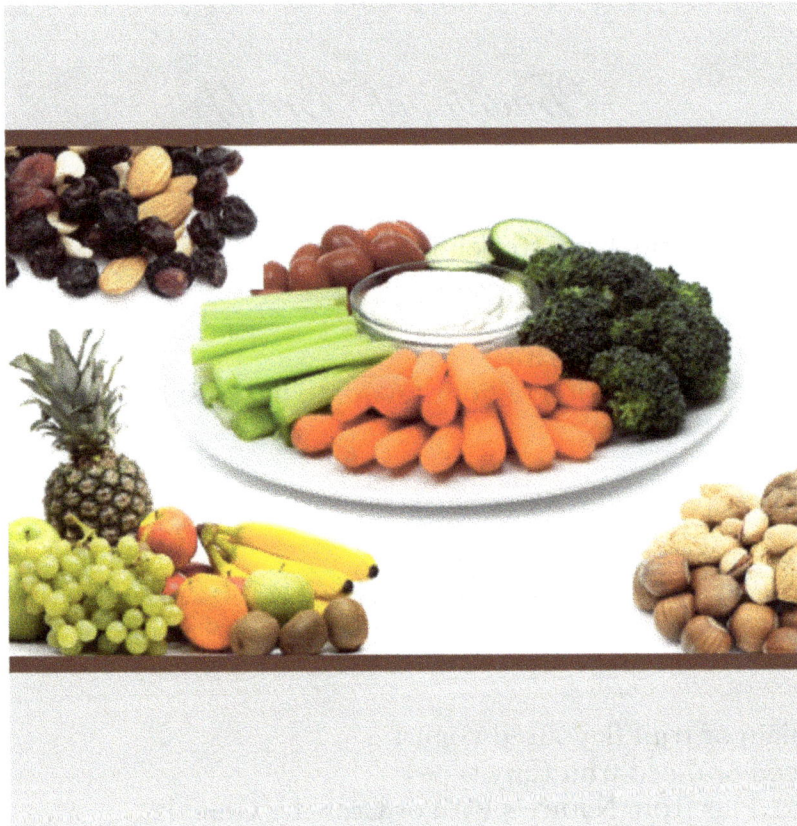

Fruit

Can be eaten; fresh, dried, or frozen

Berries
- Acai Berry
- Barberry
- Bearberry
- Blackberry
- Blueberry
- Boysenberry
- Cranberry
- Elderberry
- Gooseberry
- Grape & Raisin (dried grapes)
- June berry
- Juniper Berry
- Kiwi
- Raspberry
- Red Currant
- Salmonberry
- Sea-buckthorn Berry
- Strawberry

Citrus Fruit
- Clementine
- Grapefruit
- Kumquat
- Lemon
- Lime
- Mandarin
- Minneola Tangelo
- Orange
- Pomelo
- Sweety
- Tangerine
- Ugli

Fleshy Fruit
- Apple
- Apricot
- Avocado
- Cherry
- Dragon Fruit
- Lychee
- Mango
- Olive
- Papaya
- Peach
- Pear
- Plum
- Date
- Fig

Melons
Cantaloupe
Honeydew

Squash
Watermelon

Miscellaneous Fruit
Banana
Blackcurrant
Coconut
Crowberry

Goji Berry
Passion Fruit
Pomegranate

Multiple Fruit
Breadfruit
Custard Apple
Jackfruit

Osage-orange
Pineapple
Prune

Nuts

*Best nuts for the body
Almond*
Brazil Nut*
Cashew
Chestnut
Hazelnut

Macadamia Nut
Pine
Pistachio
Walnuts (natural parasite cleanse)

Popcorn

Eat with as little butter and salt as possible, pop yourself (no preservatives that way).

Seeds

Pumpkin (natural parasite cleans), Sunflower and Sesame

Trail Mix

Combine any type of nuts, seeds and dried fruit - maybe add a <u>few</u> carob chipits.

Vegetables & Dip

Artichoke
Asparagus
Aubergene
Beans
Beet
Broccoli
Brussels sprouts
Cabbage
Carrot
Cauliflower

Celeriac
Celery
Chard
Chicory
Collards
Corn
Cress
Cucumbers
Gourds
Jerusalem Artichoke

Kales
Kohlrabi
Leek
Lettuce
Okra is also called 'ladies' fingers' or
gumbo i
Onions
Parsnips
Peas
Peppers
Potatoes
Pumpkins
Radicchio - a chicory leaf

Radish
Rhubarb
Rutabaga
Shallots
Spinach
Squash
Swede
Sweet corn
Sweet potato
Tomatoes
Turnips
Watercress
Yams

Mushrooms - not technically a vegetable, but a far older member of the plant kingdom.
Great to cut up and to be eaten with your favourite dip recipe. *See appetizers for dip recipes.*

Lunch

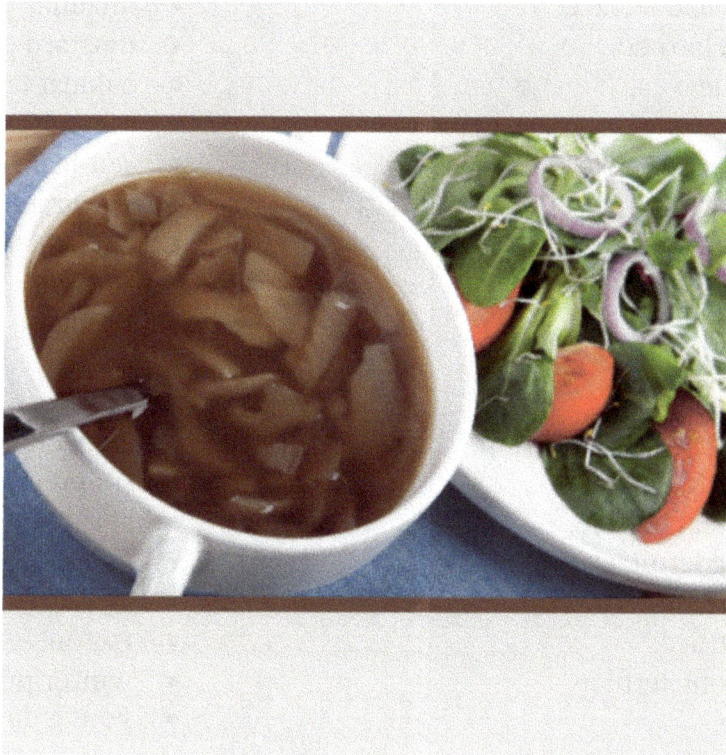

Salads

Salad Greens (your choice)

- Arugula,
- butterhead lettuce,
- Boston lettuce,
- celery leaves,
- chicory,
- chioggia,
- claytonia,
- corn salad,
- cress,
- endigia,
- escarole,
- fetticus,
- field greens,
- field lettuce,
- green leaf lettuce,
- iceberg lettuce,
- Japanese greens,
- leaf lettuce,
- limestone lettuce,
- mache,
- mediterranean rocket,
- miner's lettuce,
- mizuna,
- mustard greens,
- oakleaf lettuce,
- radicchio,
- red-leaf lettuce,
- red orach,
- red mustard,
- rocket,
- Romaine lettuce,
- roquette, rucola,
- rugola,
- spinach leaves,
- spoon cabbage,
- spring mix,
- tango,
- taratezak,
- trefoil,
- winter purslane
- young dandelion greens

BLT Chicken Club Salad

2 cooked chicken breasts
5 sliced of cooked bacon crumbled
Salt and Pepper to taste
Salad greens
2 diced tomatoes
In a large bowl combine all ingredients and stir
*See recipe for the BLT Dressing

Broccoli Salad

5 cups chopped broccoli
3 chopped green onions
1 cup halved red grapes or green grapes or raisins
¾ cup toasted almonds or sunflower seeds or pine nuts
In a large bowl combine all ingredients and stir.
*See recipe for the Broccoli Dressing

Fruit Salad

1 orange peeled & chopped
½ apple
½ pear
½ banana
½ nectarine
1/3 cup marshmallows
Optional, sprinkle of shredded coconut
In a large bowl combine all ingredients and stir.

Japanese Salad

1 small shredded head cabbage
3 cups bean sprouts
4 chopped green onions
2 cups sliced almonds
2 Tbsp sesame seeds
½ cup sliced fresh mushrooms
In a large bowl combine all ingredients and stir.
*See recipe for the Japanese Dressing

Mediterranean Salad

2 cooked breasts of chicken, sliced
3 cups shredded Salad greens
10-15 small cherry tomatoes
½ sliced cucumber
½ red bell pepper sliced thinly
10+ pitted black olives
1 small red onion sliced into smaller sections
½ cup fetta cheese
*See recipe for the Mediterranean Dressing

Roasted Chicken Caesar Salad

1 cup Salad greens
2 Tbsp Parmesan cheese
1 Tbsp Bacon bits
Tear up lettuce and combine all ingredients and stir. Serve on a plate, add Caesar dressing.

Potato Salad

9 hardboiled eggs
¾ cup mayonnaise (Hellmann's)
¾ tsp curry powder
Salt & pepper to taste
1/3 cup chopped shallots
2 lbs. yellow/gold Yukon potatoes (yellow flesh)
1-4 golden apples diced
Mash eggs & mayo, add curry, shallots, salt & pepper, mix, add apples, and potatoes. Mix.

Tossed Salad

1 cup Salad greens
Chopped vegetables of your choice
Optional: Sliced Egg, shrimp, or cooked meat
Tear up lettuce and combine all ingredients and stir. Serve on a plate with your favourite dressing on top.

Taco Salad

Cook
½ pound hamburger, cooked
1 green or red pepper cleaned and sliced
1 small chopped green onion
1 clove garlic sliced
Dash of salt & pepper
2 Tbsp soy sauce
1 Tbsp chili powder
1 Tbsp of Mexican taco dried spices
14 oz can tomato sauce

Fresh
1 cup shredded Cheddar cheese
3 cups shredded Salad greens
2 large chopped tomatoes
1 cup ranch dressing

Cook hamburger and sauté onions. Add soy sauce, tomato sauce, and spices and simmer 20 minutes.

Divide the mixture and place onto the center of the lettuce, sprinkle with cheese and add sour cream, salsa and or guacamole.

Dressings

Great on Tossed Salad
(All dressings need to be kept in the Refrigerator)

Asian Dressing

3 Tbsp of Soya Sauce
½ cup of sesame oil
Optional; add ½ tsp sesame seeds
Combine ingredients and stir.

Balsamic Vinaigrette

3 Tbsp of Balsamic Vinegar
½ cup of olive oil
Crushed garlic to taste
Salt & pepper to taste
Pinch of sugar
Combine all ingredients and stir.

Another Variation - Vinaigrette
       3 Tbsp white vinegar
       1 ½ tsp mustard
       Dash of salt & pepper
       Pinch of sugar
       ¾ cup olive oil
Combine all ingredients and stir.

BLT Dressing

       1 cup mayonnaise
       ¼ cup water
       2 Tbsp tomato paste
       1 ½ Tbsp barbeque sauce
       ½ tsp onion powder or 1 tsp onion flakes
       Dash of pepper
Combine all ingredients and stir.

Broccoli Dressing

       1 cup mayonnaise
       1 tablespoon balsamic vinegar
       1/3 cup sugar
Combine all ingredients and stir.

Caesar Dressing

1 egg chopped fine
4-5 crushed garlic cloves
1 tin anchovy chopped fine
2 Tbsp Dijon mustard
2 Tbsp lemon juice
1 dash tobacco sauce
3 dash Worcestershire sauce
1 cup olive oil
Salt & pepper to taste
Combine all ingredients and stir.

Coleslaw Dressing

2 crushed garlic cloves
2 Tbsp diced onion
½ cup lemon juice
1 tablespoon mustard
½ tsp oregano powder
1 tablespoon sugar
1 tsp salt
½ tsp pepper
¼ cup olive oil
Combine all ingredients and stir.
Shred cabbage and carrots, then pour some coleslaw dressing on top of the mix and eat.

Garlic Dressing

    2 crushed garlic cloves
    2 Tbsp fresh parsley
    1 cup cottage cheese
    ¼ cup of buttermilk (in ¼ cup put 1 tsp lemon juice, fill with milk)
    2 Tbsp vinegar
    Pinch of dried tarragon, salt, and pepper
Combine all ingredients and stir.
You may want to blend in food processor or mix very well.

Herb Dressing

    1 cup mayonnaise
    1 ½ Tbsp lemon juice
    1 tablespoon mixed herbs (Fresh-thyme, parsley & chives, or ½ tsp Mrs. Dash)
    Pinch of salt & pepper
Combine all ingredients and stir.

Italian Dressing

1 crushed garlic clove
½ cup olive oil
2 Tbsp vinegar
1 ½ tsp lemon juice
Pinch sugar
Pinch dried mustard
Pinch dried oregano
Pinch dried thyme
Pinch of dried dill
Dash of salt & pepper

Combine all ingredients and stir.
You may want to blend in food processor or mix very well.

Mediterranean Dressing

1 cup extra virgin olive oil
1/3 cup red wine vinegar
2 garlic cloves, pressed through garlic press
¼ tsp salt
1 tsp oregano, dried
½ tsp basil, dried
Juice of 1 lemon
1 tsp Dijon mustard
Add all ingredients to a jar, cover and mix well.
Use immediately and or store in the fridge.

Japanese Dressing

¼ cup vegetable spice mix
½ cup olive oil
2 Tbsp soya sauce
¼ cup vinegar
Pinch of pepper
1 tablespoon sugar
Combine all ingredients and stir.

Pesto Dressing

¾ cup fresh spinach
1 crushed garlic clove
1 ½ tablespoon olive oil
1 tablespoon lime juice
6 tablespoon parmesan cheese

Add first four ingredients in food processor and blend add cheese and stir. Or mix very well until mixture becomes creamy and smooth.

Soups

Borscht

¼ cup butter
¼ onion diced
Salt and pepper to taste
2 carrots shredded
10 large potato shredded
2 beets shredded
Water (approximately 2 inches over veggies)
1 Small cabbage shredded (4-5 cups)
1 medium tomato diced
1 can tomato
1 cup cream
½ tsp dill

In a big pot on medium heat, mix butter & onion, add salt & pepper, carrots, potatoes & beets, boil all vegetables in the water for 10 minutes, add all other ingredients and simmer for 1 hour. Remove from heat and serve.

Beef Barley Soup

1 lb steak, cubed small
3 qtrs. water
1 ½ stalks celery, diced
2 ½ cups carrots, diced
1 medium onion diced
1/3 cup pearl barley
3-6 Tbsp liquid bouillon (beef)
¾ cups peas (frozen)
1 ½ cups potatoes, diced

Sauté beef in 2 Tbsp olive oil. In a big pot bring water to boil. Add all vegetables and boil until tender. Add beef bouillon. Simmer 15 minutes. Remove from heat and serve.

Chicken Soup

3 qtrs. water
2 chicken breasts cubed
1 cup celery, chopped
1 small onion chopped, chopped
1 cup carrots, diced
½ cup peas
3 Tbsp liquid bouillon (chicken)
2 Tbsp dry bouillon (chicken)
½ tsp of salt,

In large pot bring salted water to a boil. Add all ingredients and simmer until tender. Remove from heat and serve.
For Chicken Rice Soup – add ¼ cup rice

Cream of Broccoli Soup

3 qtrs. water
¾ cups celery (finely minced)
1 small onion chopped (finely minced)
2 large heads of fresh broccoli, cut up (or 1 kg frozen)
2 Tbsp carrots (finely grated)
3 Tbsp liquid bouillon (chicken)
2 Tbsp dry bouillon (chicken)
½ cup evaporated milk
¼ cup cheese whiz
½ tsp of salt,
¼ tsp baking soda (prevents curdling)
6 Tbsp corn starch, stirred into ½ cup water

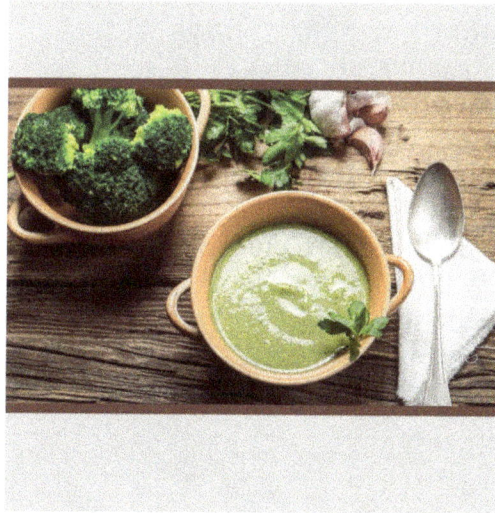

In large pot bring salted water to a boil. Add all vegetables and simmer until tender. Add bouillon. Use potato masher to further breakdown broccoli. Add cheese whiz. Stir until completely blended. Add baking soda. Stir well. Add milk. Stir until gently boiling. Thicken with cornstarch to desired consistency. Remove from heat and serve.

Cream of Mushroom Soup

¼ cup butter
¾ lb mushrooms, sliced
3 qtrs. water
1 small onion chopped (finely chopped)
½ stock celery (finely chopped)
1 Tbsp carrot, grated
3 Tbsp liquid bouillon (chicken)
6 Tbsp dry bouillon (chicken)
½ cup evaporated milk
¼ tsp baking soda (prevents curdling)
6 Tbsp corn starch, stirred into ½ cup water

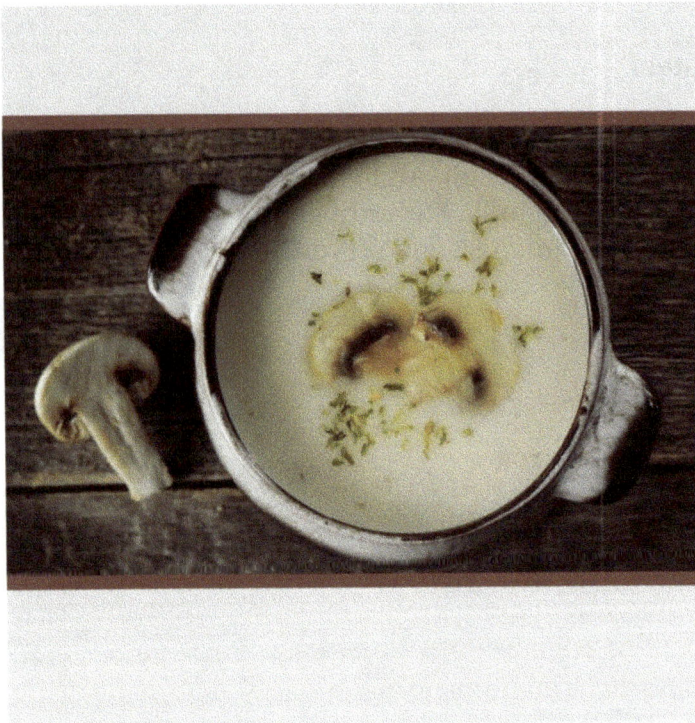

In large pot sauté mushrooms in butter, add water and bring to a boil. Add all vegetables and bring back to a boil. Add bouillon. Stir until completely blended. Add baking soda. Stir well. Add milk. Stir until gently boiling. Thicken with cornstarch to desired consistency. Bring to gentle boil, then remove from heat and serve.

Seafood Chowder

1 tsp butter
¼ onion diced
2 green onion chopped
3 large mushrooms diced
> In large pot sauté onions, butter, and mushrooms.
¼ cup water
½ red pepper diced
4 stakes celery diced
4 med potatoes diced
1 carrot diced
1 tsp salt
1 tsp pepper
2 garlic cloves diced
1 tsp parsley
¼ tsp Cajun pepper
1 tsp Mrs. Dash Spice
> Add ¼ cup water, red pepper, celery, potatoes, carrot, and spice cut for another 5 minutes.
¾ cups water
15-20 shrimp cut in half
1 can real crab drained
2 cans clams drained
1 bag frozen scallops
3 cups milk
¼ cup cream
1 can mushroom soup

¼ cup parmesan cheese

¼ cup cheddar cheese

> ➤ Add remainder of ingredients, stir and boil for 5 minutes.
> ➤ Turn down heat and simmer for 20 minutes.

Remove from heat and serve.

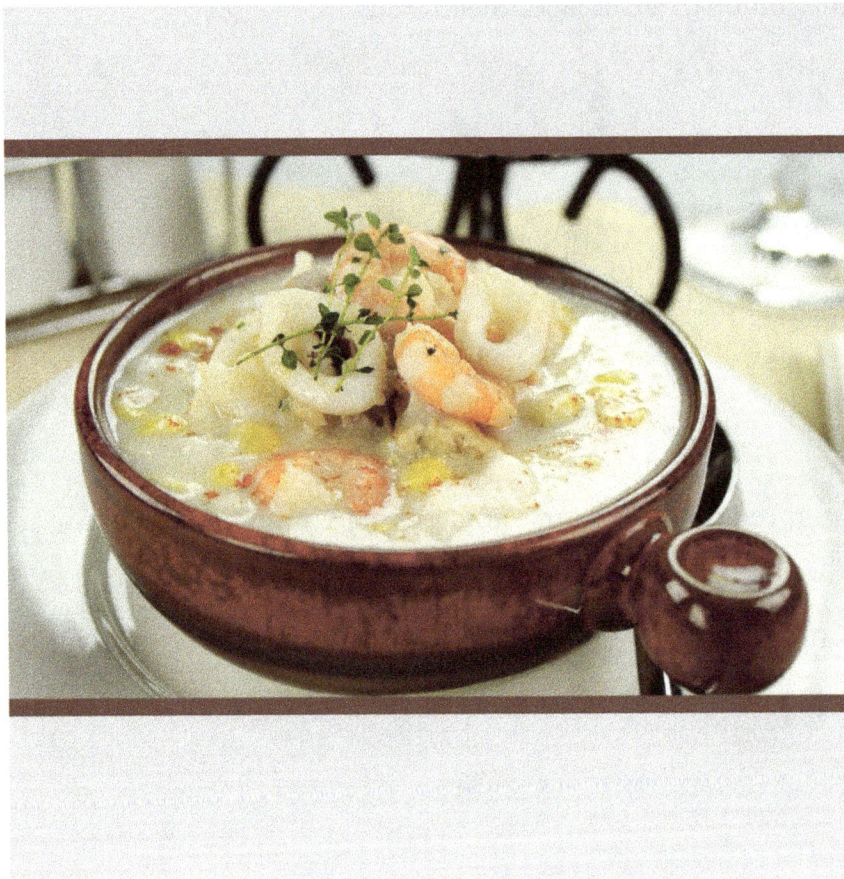

Turkey Soup

Cook turkey and pick meat from bones. In Dutch oven size pot, boil bones for 2 hours (4-5 qtrs. water). Strain liquid, throw away the bones and return liquid to pot.

Add
2 celery stalks, chopped
1 small onion, diced
1 ½ cups carrots, diced
¾ cups frozen peas
2 cups potatoes, diced
½ tsp basil
2 tsp salt
Optional, 2-3 Tbsp liquid bouillon (chicken)
Bring water to boil. Add all vegetables and diced turkey Simmer until tender, remove from heat and serve.

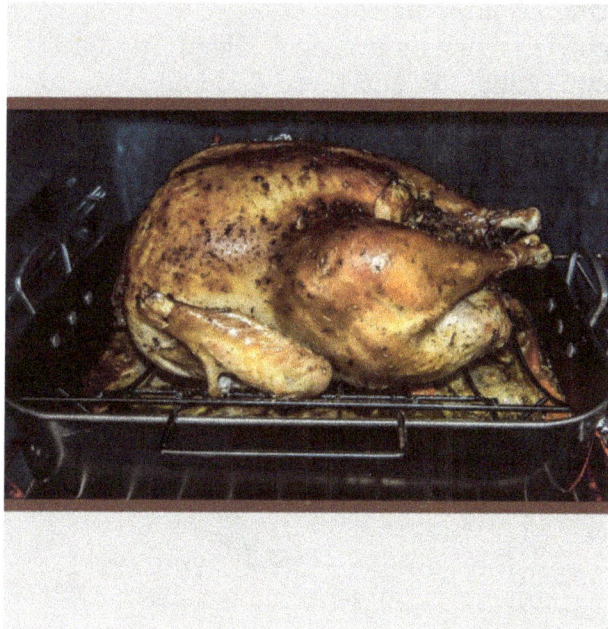

Vegetable Soup

3 qtrs. water
2 celery stalks, chopped
¼ cup green pepper cleaned and chopped
1 cup green beans, chopped
3 large mushrooms, chopped
1 medium onion, diced
1 ½ cups carrots, quartered & sliced
1 ½ cups zucchini, quartered & sliced
14 oz can dice tomatoes
¾ tsp fennel
½ tsp basil
4 Tbsp liquid bouillon (veggie)
½ tsp salt
¼ tsp pepper

Bring water to boil. Add all vegetables and tomato. Return to boil. Add spices and bouillon. Simmer until celery is very tender, remove from heat and serve.

Meat and Vegetable Soup

Same as vegetable soup, but add 1 cup of your favourite pre-cooked meat cubed and onions. Then add vegetables and spices, fill with water until it covers all ingredients. Cook on medium for ¾ hour or until all ingredients are tender.

Lettuce Wraps

Chicken Fajita

2 chicken breasts sliced into thin strips, cooked
1 zucchini sliced diagonally
1 green or red pepper cleaned and sliced
1 small onion thinly sliced
1 clove garlic sliced
Dash of salt & pepper
1 package of Mexican fajita dried spices
¼ cup (1 oz) shredded Cheddar cheese
2 large lettuce leaves or shredded as salad

Cook chicken and sauté onions, red pepper, garlic, and zucchini. Add spices and stir for 2 minutes longer.

Divide the mixture and place onto the center of the lettuce, sprinkle with cheese and add sour cream, salsa and or guacamole.

Fold the lettuce into a wrap and eat.

Rice Wrap (s)

ASIAN WRAP

¼ cup cooked protein (chicken)
½ cup cooked rice
½ to 1 tsp red onion
1 Tbsp peanuts
½ tsp soya sauce
2 Tbsp chopped spinach
2 large lettuce leaves

CARAMELIZED ONION WRAP

¼ cup cooked protein (chicken, turkey, beef, shrimp, or pork. etc.)
½ cup cooked rice
2 Tbsp shredded carrot
1 Tbsp red ginger slaw
1 tsp caramelized onions
1 tsp to 1 Tbsp teriyaki sauce
2 large lettuce leaves

CHICKEN RANCH WRAP

¼ cup cooked protein (chicken)
½ cup cooked rice
2 Tbsp shredded cheese
1 tsp to 1 Tbsp ranch dressing
2 large lettuce leaves

GREEK WRAP

¼ cup cooked protein (chicken, turkey, beef, lamb, shrimp, or pork. etc.)
½ cup cooked rice
1 Tbsp shredded cucumber
1 Tbsp chopped tomato (optional, sliced olives)
1 Tbsp feta cheese
½ to 1 tsp red onion
½ to 1 Tbsp tzatziki sauce
2 large lettuce leaves

ITALIAN WRAP

¼ cup cooked protein (ground beef)
½ cup cooked rice
1 tsp chopped celery
1 tsp chopped onions
1 tsp to 1 Tbsp tomato sauce
Sprinkle ¼ to ½ tsp oregano or Italian spices
2 large lettuce leaves

PIZZA WRAP

¼ cup cooked protein (pepperoni, chicken, ham & pineapple, or shrimp & mushroom, etc.)
½ cup cooked rice
1 tsp chopped cooked or raw veggies (onions, green peppers, tomatoes, etc.)
1 tsp to 1 Tbsp pizza sauce or barbeque sauce
2 Tbsp shredded cheese
Sprinkle ¼ to ½ tsp oregano
2 large lettuce leaves

SHRIMP WRAP

¼ to ½ cup cooked protein (shrimp)
½ cup cooked rice
1 Tbsp chopped green bell pepper
1 Tbsp chopped snow peas
2 Tbsp chopped spinach
1 tsp to 1 Tbsp garlic mayo
2 large lettuce leaves

THAI WRAP

¼ cup cooked protein (chicken, turkey, beef, shrimp, or pork. etc.)
½ cup cooked rice
2 Tbsp shredded cucumber
1 Tbsp red ginger slaw
½ to 1 tsp peanut sauce
2 large lettuce leaves

WESTERN WRAP

¼ to ½ cup cooked protein (scrambled eggs & bacon)
½ cup hash browns
1 Tbsp chopped green bell pepper
1 tsp chopped onions
2 Tbsp chopped spinach
2 Tbsp shredded cheese
1 tsp to 1 Tbsp salsa
1 tsp to 1 Tbsp chipotle mayo
2 large lettuce leaves

Taco Wrap

½ pound hamburger, cooked
1 green or red pepper cleaned and sliced
1 small onion thinly sliced
1 clove garlic sliced
Dash of salt & pepper
1 Tbsp of Mexican taco dried spices
¼ cup (1 oz) shredded Cheddar cheese
2 large lettuce leaves (or shredded as salad)

Cook hamburger and sauté onions, red pepper, and garlic. Add spices and stir for 2 minutes longer. Divide the mixture and place onto the center of the lettuce, sprinkle with cheese and add sour cream, salsa and or guacamole. Fold the lettuce into a wrap and eat.

Tuna Salad Wrap

Great for lunch. Makes two full sandwiches
1 celery stick finely chopped
1 tablespoon chopped onion
1 diced pickle
250 ml can Tuna (drain)
2 Tbsp Mayonnaise
¼ tsp salt
¼ tsp pepper
¼ cup (1 oz) shredded Cheddar cheese
2 large lettuce leaves

Cut up first two ingredients and place into a small bowl. Combine drained tuna, mayonnaise, salt and pepper Stir. Divide the mixture in the bowl into two and place each half onto the center of the lettuce.

Add shredded cheese on top. Fold the lettuce into a wrap and eat.

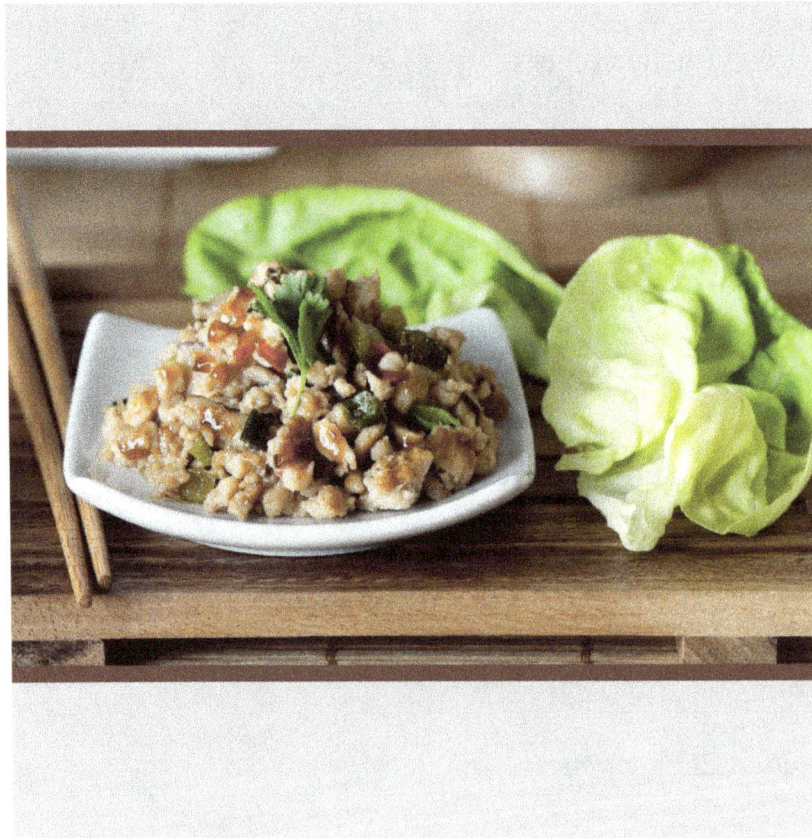

Appetizers

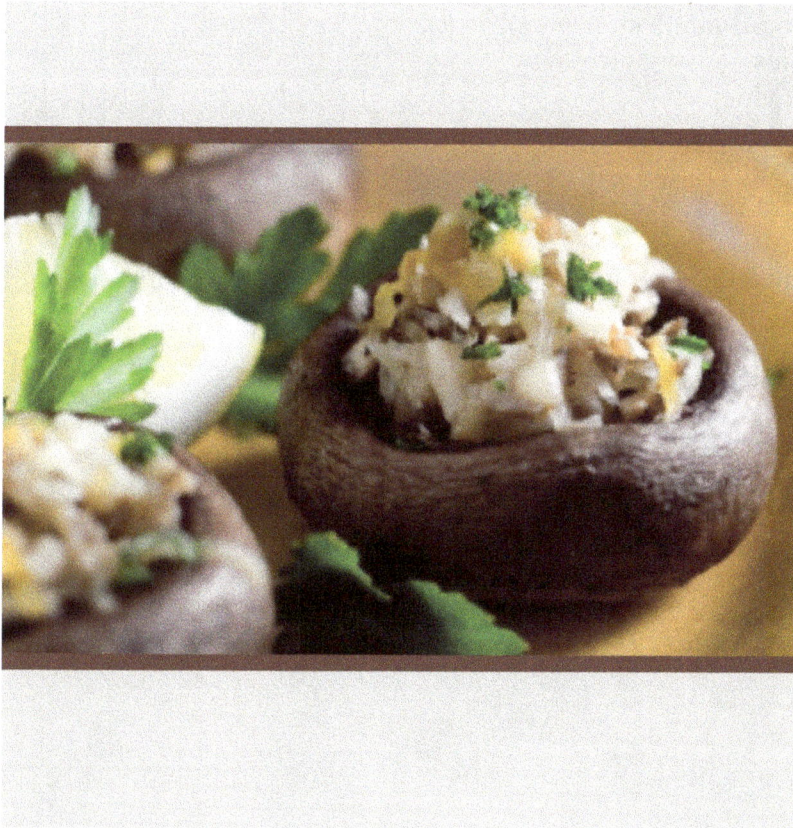

Antipasto

1 green bell pepper diced
1 red bell pepper diced
1 can sliced mushrooms
1 lb cauliflower
1 small jar of tiny onions
1 32 oz jar of dill pickles
1 tin anchovies
½ cup white vinegar
30 oz ketchup (3 ¾ cups)
½ cup olive oil
2 tins tuna, drained
1 can crabmeat
Chop into small bit size, heat to boil, stirring. Put into 6 pint canning jars & process 30 minutes.

Celery Sticks

- With Hummus
- Peanut Butter
- Cheese
- Dip

Crackers

Serves 6

    1 cup buckwheat grouts
    1 cup sunflower seeds
    ½ cup flaxseeds
    ½ cup water
    4 Tbsp agave nectar or honey
    Dash of salt & pepper
    2 Tbsp lemon juice

Soak buckwheat grouts for 30 minutes in water. Rinse and drain.
Soak sunflower seeds for 1 hour in water. Rinse and drain.
Soak flaxseed for 30 minutes in ½ cup water. Do not drain.
In food processor, grind all ingredients until chunky.
Spread on dehydrator trays with non-stick sheets or use parchment paper (cut out a hole).
You can pre-cut into squares or break into chunks once dried.
Dehydrate at 145° for 2 hours and then 110° for 12 hours or until crunchy.

Or Crackers made from Almonds
Serves 4

    2 cup almonds
    ½ cup flaxseeds or Red River
    ½ tsp salt
    2 Tbsp lemon juice

Soak the almonds for 12 hours in water. Rinse and drain.
Grind flaxseeds to a powder in coffee grinder.
In food processor, grind almonds, flaxseeds, salt and lemon juice, until smooth.
Spread on dehydrator trays with non-stick sheets or use parchment paper (cut out a hole).
Dehydrate at 115° for 24 hours

Put Sliced Meat, Cheese, Pickles,
Tomatoes, or Avocado on the crackers

Pickles - Dill

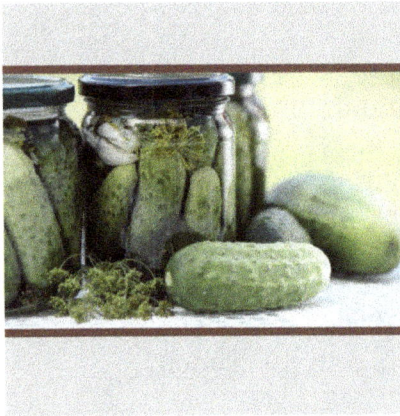

Vinegar Mixture
3 qtrs. water (12 cups)
1 cup coarse salt
3 cups vinegar
➤ Boil 2 min,
Kirby or English cucumbers

Remove hot jars from canner. Place 1 head fresh dill or 1 tsp (5 mL) dill seeds and 1 clove garlic into each jar; pack in cucumbers.

Pour boiling vinegar mixture over cucumbers to within ½ inch (1 cm) of rim (head space). Put lids on. Place back in the canner and process 10 minutes for pint (500 mL) jars and 15 minutes for quart (1 L) jars

Optional - Can carrots, asparagus, tiny onions, (or boiled eggs with a few sliced red onion).

Stuffed Eggs

6 hard boiled eggs
¼ cup mayonnaise
Dash of salt and pepper
¼ cup finely chopped onion
Optional: 1 -2 tsp horseradish
or ½ tsp hot pepper sauce
Optional: 3 Tbsp pre-cooked bacon bits
Paprika to garnish

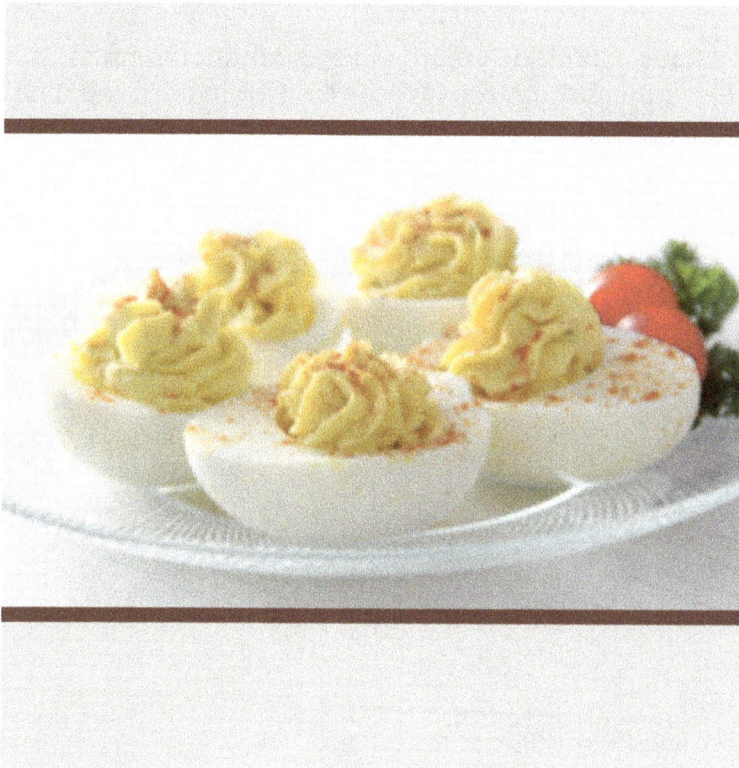

Peel and cut eggs in half. Scrape cooked yoke out and mash in a bowl. Stir in mayonnaise, onions, and spices. Spoon into hallowed out egg whites. Sprinkle paprika on top as garnish. Refrigerate until ready to eat.

There are special egg plates you can purchase to hold eggs up right.

Stuffed Mushrooms

Makes 20   400° 25 Minutes

20 medium mushrooms
6 Tbsp butter
1 - 8-oz package cream cheese, softened
¼ cup finely chopped onion
2 Tbsp of Ranch or Knorr vegetable spice dip mix
Optional: 1 can (approx. 120g) of crab and or shrimp (drained)
Optional: 3 Tbsp pre-cooked bacon bits
½ cup of grated cheese (mozzarella, cheddar, mix)

Remove stems from mushrooms, chop stems. Combine cream cheese, onion, chopped mushroom stems, ranch mix and stir. Place mushroom caps whole side up in a baking dish. Fill mushroom caps with mixture. Sprinkle cheese on top. Place in oven and bake.

Walnuts

1 egg white
1 tsp cold water
  ➤ Beat egg and water until bubbly,
1 cup brown sugar
1 ¼ tsp salt
  ➤ Mix in a separate bowl
4 cups halved walnuts
  ➤ Put walnuts into egg solution
  ➤ Then in sugar (coat completely)
  ➤ Bake for ½ to ¾ hour at 250° (Check often)

Dips

Guacamole

2-3 ripe avocados or 10 ozs cooked chopped asparagus
2 tsp lime juice
1 ½ tsp onion powder <u>or</u> ½ cup diced onions
½ tsp garlic powder <u>or</u> 1 tsp minced garlic
¼ tsp Mexican <u>or</u> black pepper
¼ tsp salt
Dash of Cilantro or 2 Tbsp of chopped leaves
Dash of hot pepper sauce <u>or</u> pinch of cayenne pepper
1/3 cup peeled seeded chopped & drained tomato
3 Tbsp chopped green chillies (remove stems and seeds)

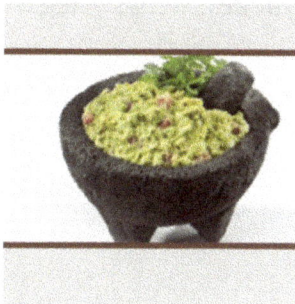

Place in blender and blend or mash with wooden spoon; avocado or asparagus, lime, onion, garlic, pepper, salt, cilantro, and hot pepper sauce.
Stir in tomatoes and green chillies.
Serve as dip with nut crackers, fresh vegetables or on top of taco / fajita meat salad.

Secret to the avocado dip turning brown; place whole avocado seed(s) back into bowl and serve.

Herb Dip

1 cup cream cheese
1 cup plain yogurt or sour cream
3 Tbsp mayonnaise
8 Tbsp sliced green onions
2 Tbsp chopped chives
½ tsp mustard
Dash of hot pepper sauce
Combine and blend well: cream cheese, yogurt, and mayonnaise. Mix in remaining ingredients. Refrigerate two hours to overnight. Serve with raw vegetables.

Honey Mustard Dip

½ cup honey
½ cup sour cream or plain yogurt
¼ cup mayonnaise
2 Tbsp mustard
Combine all ingredients and mix until smooth. Eat with vegetables or chicken wings / legs.

Mustard Dip

8 ozs cream cheese
½ cup sour cream
2 Tbsp mustard
Combine all ingredients and mix until smooth. Eat with vegetables or chicken wings/legs.

Mexican Bean Dip

1 can of refried beans
1 ½ tsp onion powder
½ tsp garlic powder
3 Tbsp chopped green chillies
Dash of Hot pepper sauce
1½ tsp chili powder
¼ cup chopped green onion
¼ cup chopped green or red pepper
¾ cup mayonnaise
¾ cup plain yogurt or sour cream
2 tablespoon Mexican seasoning (taco or fajita)
1 can sliced olives, drained
1 cup shredded cheddar cheese
Combine refried beans, hot pepper sauce, chilli powder. Spread on 10-inch cookie sheet.
Sprinkle with onion and green peppers. In a bowl stir together mayonnaise, sour cream
Mexican spice; spread on top of green peppers. Sprinkle with olives and cheddar cheese.
Cover and chill for 3-5 hours to overnight.

Serve as dip with nut crackers, fresh vegetables or on top of taco / fajita meat salad.

Nut Dip

½ cup pine nuts
1 cup hazelnuts
¼ cup olive oil
½ tsp salt
2 Tbsp lemon juice
1 crushed garlic clove
Combine all and grind in food processor,
Add ½ cup fresh basil, chopped and stir

Salsa

4 ripe tomatoes, finely chopped
4 cloves garlic, minced
¾ white onion, finely chopped
1/3 each green, red and orange bell pepper, seeded and chopped
2 Tbsp. chopped fresh cilantro
1 Tbsp. ground cumin,
2 ½ tsp lemon juice
2 tsp salt & 1 tsp ground black pepper
Option #1 – for hot salsa add 1 jalapeno pepper, 1 serrano pepper, seeded and chopped
Option #2 – exchange the cumin for
- 1 Tbsp. balsamic vinegar
- ½ tsp basil
- ½ tsp oregano
Combine all ingredients

Tzatziki Dip

The only trick is to properly drain the cucumber before mixing it into the yogurt.

2 cups grated well drained cucumber (from about 1 medium 10-oz English cucumber, no need to peel or seed the cucumber first, grate on the large holes of your box grater)
1 ½ cups plain Greek yogurt
2 Tbsp extra-virgin olive oil
2 Tbsp chopped fresh mint and or dill
1 tablespoon lemon juice
1 medium clove garlic, pressed or minced
½ tsp fine sea salt

Lightly squeeze the grated cucumber between your palms over the sink to remove excess moisture (place a strainer underneath to catch anything that falls but will still let the moisture out) or use a cheese cloth. Transfer the squeezed cucumber to a serving bowl and repeat with the remaining cucumber.

For best results, combine all the ingredients except for the cucumber and dill, then let it rest overnight in the fridge while your cucumber is draining.

Add the yogurt, olive oil, herbs, lemon juice, garlic, and salt to the bowl, and stir to blend. Let the mixture rest for 5 minutes to allow the flavors to meld. Taste and add additional chopped fresh herbs, lemon juice, and or salt, if necessary.

Taco Dip

Bottom layer – 1 can refried beans
Next layer – 2 med avocados, mashed
Next layer – Tomatoes & olives, diced
Next layer – 3 Tbsp taco spice mixed in small container of sour cream
Top layer – shredded 'Tex Mex' Cheese

Vegetable Spinach Dip

8 ozs or 1 cup of frozen spinach (double if fresh)
1 cup plain yogurt or sour cream
¾ cup mayonnaise
¼ cup vegetable dried spice (Knorr, Watkins, or Ranch)
2 tsp parsley
1 tsp garlic powder
¼ green onions

Optional - add a can of shrimp or crab or both

If using frozen spinach, thaw, and squeeze until dry. In medium bowl stir all ingredients together. Cover and refrigerate for two hours. Serve with nut crackers or fresh vegetables.

Dinner

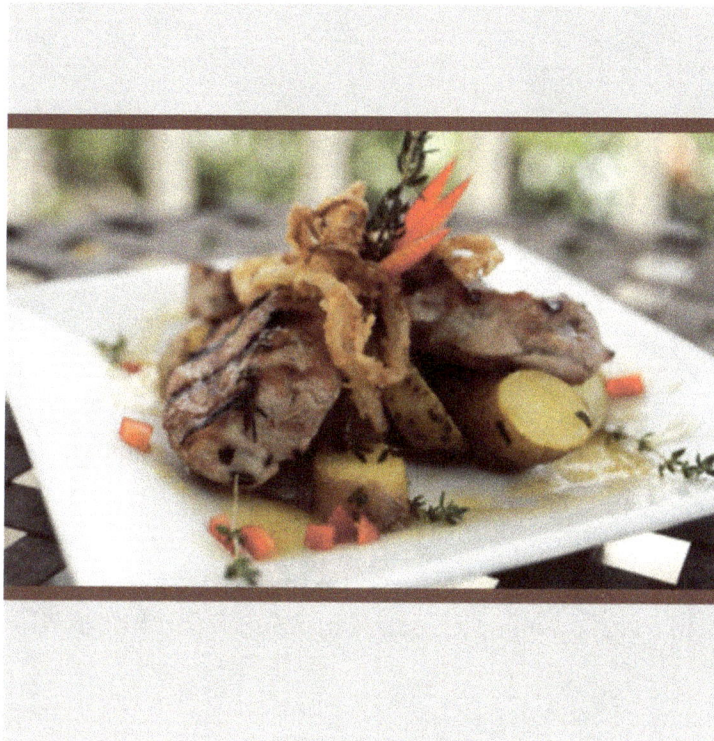

Barbeque Sauce

1 cup chili sauce
1 cup President's choice beer & chipotle BBQ sauce
½ cup brown sugar
¼ lemon juice
1 tsp mustard powder
Mix together

Barbeque Ribs

Cut pork back ribs (or side ribs) into smaller serving size (3-4 ribs, or half rack).
Cut aluminum foil into pieces that are big enough to wrap the ribs.
Coat the ribs generously with sauce and wrap them with foil. Marinate in the fridge overnight.

Remove from the fridge about an hour before cooking (to bring to room temperature).
Bake the wrapped ribs in oven on a cookie sheet at 350° F for 1 hour, then reduce heat to 275° for another hour.

There is enough sauce to do about 2-3 serving sizes.

Beef Stew

1-pound cubed beef (steak), browned
1 tsp bacon bits
3 cups Water
Pinch of salt & pepper
1 small onion diced
3 potatoes diced or cubed
1 carrot sliced
½ peas

Brown beef, add onions & bacon bits, mix 2 minutes, add water, simmer two hours. Add all other ingredients boil 45 minutes to 1 hour (Until potatoes are cooked).

Chili

1 pound of hamburger, browned
1 slice bacon, cut up
Pinch of salt & pepper
1 small onion
½ red pepper, cleaned and diced
3 celery sticks, chopped
2 cans of Brown beans
1 can of Kidney beans, drained
2 Tbsp sugar
1 tablespoon vinegar
1 tablespoon chili powder
1 tsp garlic powder

On stove top in large pot brown hamburger, salt and pepper, cook bacon, sauté onions, red pepper and celery. Add bean, sugar, vinegar, chilli and garlic powder, cook on medium heat 15 minutes then simmer for 1 to 1 ½ hours.

Spaghetti Squash - Baked

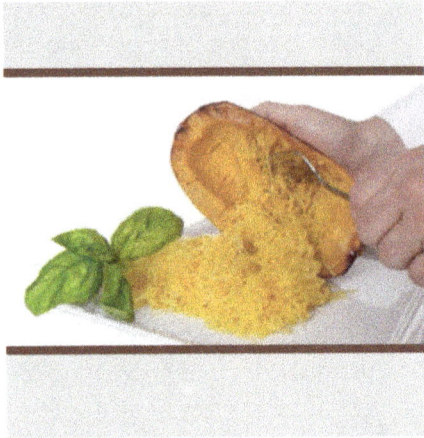

Oven 350 ° F (170 C)   30 minutes

Makes 2-3 servings

1 medium spaghetti squash halved and cleaned of seeds
2-3 cups water
1 tablespoon of butter
½ tsp salt
½ tsp black pepper
¼ cup of grated Parmesan cheese
½ tsp basil
½ cup of shredded mozzarella cheese
¼ cup of grated Parmesan cheese

Place spaghetti squash cut side up in a 10"x15" (4L) casserole dish. Add 1 inch of water to the bottom of the dish (like it is floating on water). Sprinkle parmesan cheese in the squash halves. Dot with the butter, seasoning, salt, and pepper. Bake in center of the oven for 30 minutes or until squash is tender. Scoop the spaghetti-like flesh out of the skin and place in a large bowl. Toss with basil and remaining cheese.

Note- you can cook the halved squash in the microwave by itself for 20 minutes.

Spaghetti - Vegetable

SAUTÉED MIXED VEGETABLES
WITH SPAGHETTI SQUASH

Cooked Spaghetti squash
3 Tbsp extra-virgin olive oil
½ cup chopped onions
1 lb. zucchini, diced
1 lb. broccoli florets, chopped
2 red peppers, diced
6 mushrooms, sliced
¼ tsp salt
Freshly ground black pepper to taste
½ cup shredded basil
½ cup chopped Italian or broad-leaf parsley
¼ cup grated Parmesan cheese

Cook Spaghetti squash (see recipe).
Heat oil in skillet over medium heat. Add onions and sauté until wilted, about 10 minutes.
Add other vegetables and cook, stirring occasionally, until cooked but still firm, about 7
minutes more. Add salt, pepper, basil, and parsley and mix well.
Toss spaghetti squash and vegetables, top with grated cheese, and serve.

*You can vary this recipe by using any number of seasonal vegetables, including cauli-
flower, green beans, peas, zucchini, or yellow squash - even cucumber. In place of the
Parmesan cheese, stir in 8 ozs of chèvre, or soft goat cheese, before adding basil and
seasoning to taste.

Spaghetti Squash Vegetable Pesto

Cooked Spaghetti squash
2 cups loosely packed fresh basil leaves
½ cup pine nuts or broken walnuts cup
½ cup grated Parmesan cheese
2 cloves garlic, chopped
½ cup extra-virgin olive oil
2 Tbsp olive oil
2 lb. asparagus, cut into ½ inch lengths
½ lb. green beans cut into ½ inch lengths

Cook Spaghetti squash (see recipe)
To make pesto, place fresh basil, pine nuts, Parmesan cheese, and chopped garlic in blender or food processor. With motor running, slowly add olive oil, adding more if needed, and purée. When smooth, set aside.
Heat olive oil in skillet over medium-low heat and sauté asparagus and beans, stirring occasionally, until cooked but not limp, about 10 minutes. Add 1 cup pesto, stir thoroughly, and cook until heated through.
Toss spaghetti squash with vegetables and pesto and serve.

* For variety, substitute one cup of yogurt for the pesto and sprinkle with chopped almonds or with toasted sesame seeds.

Substitute ½ pound cubed zucchini for either the asparagus or the beans. The pesto recipe makes ample portions; refrigerate leftover pesto for another use.

Spaghetti Meatballs

½ pound hamburger
¼ cup cheese (cheddar, or your choice)
¼ onion, diced
3 mushrooms, chopped
1 egg
¼ cup sauce (mushroom or spaghetti)
Salt and pepper to taste

In a bowl combine all the ingredients.
Take a small amount and roll into a ball in the palm of your hand. Makes approximately 12.
Place on greased baking sheet. Continue until all of the ingredients are rolled. Place in oven at 350 ° F for about 30 -40 minutes (depending on how well you like your hamburger cooked).
Remove from oven and eat with spaghetti or potatoes.

MEAT LOAF – place mixed ingredients into a cake pan and place in oven for about the same amount of time. Remove, cut into portions, and serve.

Spaghetti Sauce

1 lb of hamburger
1 slice of bacon cut up
½ tsp salt
½ tsp black pepper
¼ chopped onion
1 chopped green or red pepper
Hand full of fresh spinach
5 large chopped mushrooms
2 stalks of celery chopped
One jar of favourite spaghetti sauce (or make your own)

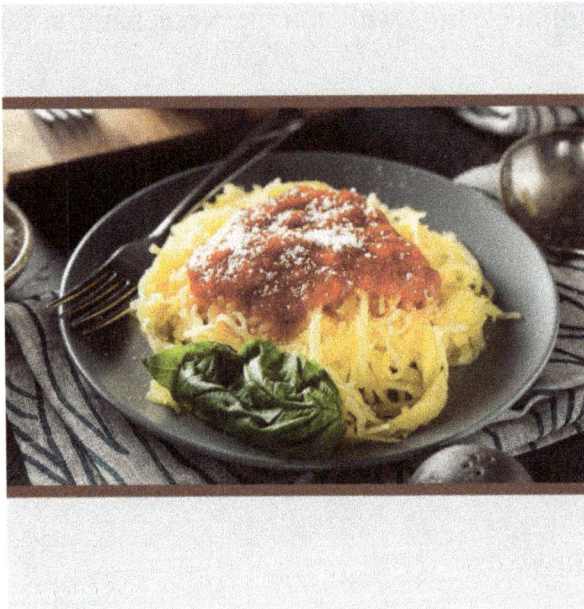

In a fry pan, brown hamburger meat and bacon on high. Lower temperature to medium and add salt and pepper, Onions, Peppers, Spinach, Mushrooms and Celery.

Cook until soft about eight - ten minutes. Add spaghetti sauce heat for additional 5 minutes. Pour onto Spaghetti squash top with cheese. Some people like to add a tablespoon of sour cream. Enjoy!

Meat

BEEF, CHICKEN, FISH, HAM, OR PORK
Oven, pan fried or barbequed

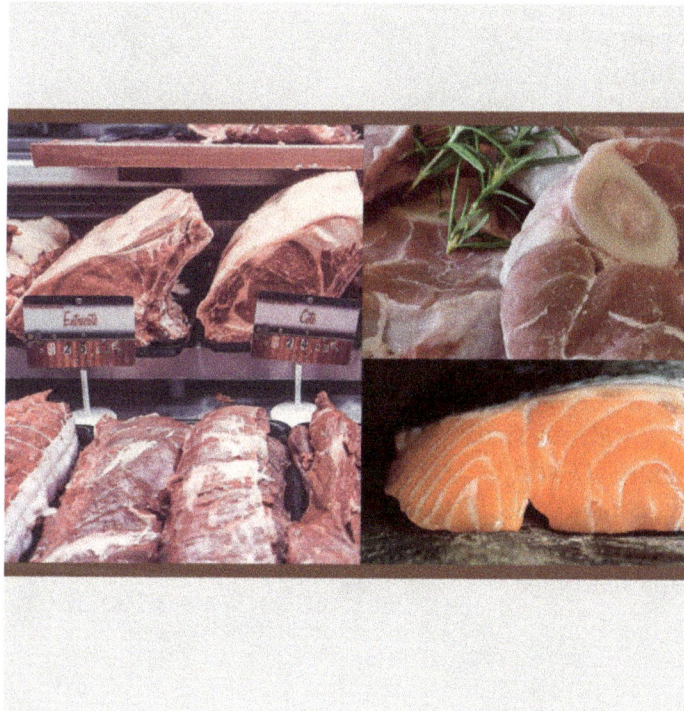

Beef - Steak

Use your favorite cut, barbeque sauce, and Spices

Pierce steak with a fork. Coat the steak with barbeque sauce and spices. Marinate steak for ½ hour to overnight in sealed container.

Heat pan or if using grilling equipment; use butter spray to coat metal. Cook steak 8-10 minutes / side. Remove from heat and place on plate and let sit for 2-4 minutes and then place on new plate and serve.

Optional: Neptune Topping
¼ cup chopped green onion
2 Tbsp butter
8 ozs cream cheese
1 tablespoon fresh garlic
2 cups crab and or shrimp
 Sliced mushrooms
2 Tbsp of parsley
¼ cup parmesan
1 tsp dill weed

Sauté onions and pepper in butter, add milk and cream cheese till melted. Add mushrooms, spice and seafood. Cook until mushrooms are tender. Spoon over steak and sprinkle with parmesan cheese.

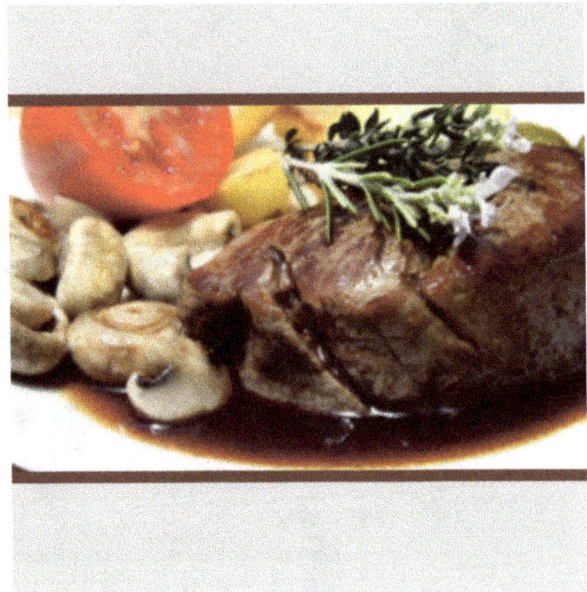

Whole Roasted Beef

Roast
Chopped Potatoes (optional-peeled)
Sliced Carrots
Diced Onions
Whole Mushrooms
¼ tsp salt
¼ tsp black pepper

Pre-heat oven, 450 °
Put roast in casserole or roasting pan.
Add ½" to 1" of water in bottom of the pan.
Add potatoes, carrots, onions, and mushrooms around the roast. Sprinkle salt and pepper on top. Cover and place in oven and cook for 45 minutes.
Remove from oven and pan and slice up meat.
Place on a plate and serve.

I must tell you a story... This newly wed couple was enjoying the bliss of matrimony. One day the young man came home to find his new bride using one of the wedding gifts, an impressive roasting pan. He was intrigued on how his wife cut off both ends of the roast and then proceeded to put it into the pan. He asked her, "Hon, why do you throw away the ends of the roast?" And she answered, "That is how my mother and grandmother cook a roast."
At the next family get together he politely asked his new mother-in-law the same question, "Why do you throw away the ends of the roast?" His mother-in=law answered, "Because that is how you cook a roast."
From the end of the dinner table you could her a chuckle coming from the grandmother, "Ah, I only cooked a roast that way because your grandfather was so cheap, he wouldn't buy me a bigger roasting pan."

Barbequed Chicken

Chicken breast, legs, or wings, sprinkled with barbeque sauce, salt, pepper and or spice.
Place onto heated barbeque.
Cook approximately 10 minutes per side.

Chicken Kabobs

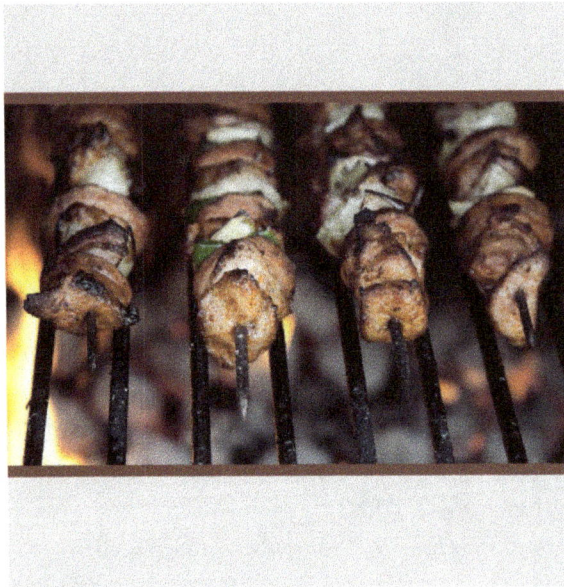

Chicken
Mushrooms
Onion
Pineapple

Using a wood spear, alternate ingredients on skewer. Brush on barbeque sauce.
Grill for 10 -15 minutes, turning occasionally.

Chicken, Rice, and Cashew Casserole

2 ½ cups 1-inch cubed cooked chicken

2 cups cooked rice (wild, basmati, or jasmine)

1 cup salted whole cashews

1 cup (2 stalks) celery, sliced

¼ cup uncooked long grain rice

¼ cup fresh parsley, chopped (or 2 Tbsp of dried)

3 Tbsp melted butter

2 cups chicken broth

2 red peppers, chopped

1 cup sour cream

1 tsp dried basil leaves

½ tsp salt

2 tsp chopped fresh garlic

Heat Oven to 350 °.

In casserole or 13 x 9" baking pan stir all ingredients together, cover.

Bake 40 minutes, stirring occasionally until rice is tender.

Uncover, continue baking for another 10 to 15 minutes, or until rice has absorbed all liquid.

Pan Fried Chicken

4 -6 Chicken Breasts
2 Tbsp butter (or ¼ cup of water)
1 small onion (or 3 green onions, chopped)
6 Mushrooms, sliced
¼ tsp black pepper
¼ tsp salt (optional, other spices)
Optional, garlic

Using a large frying pan and melt the butter or heat the water. Put the chicken into the pan. Allow them to fry for a few moments and then turn them over. Add onions, mushrooms, salt, pepper, and spices.

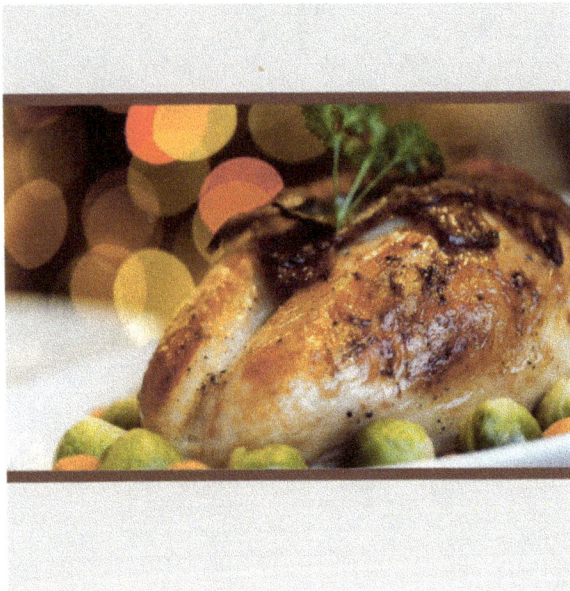

Cook on the stove top on Med/high for 35 – 45 minutes or until all pink is gone from the meat. Remove from pan and place on a plate and serve.

Chicken Fingers
Oven Roasted Chicken

12 -18 pieces of chicken legs, or four breasts, sliced
½ cup of barbeque sauce
Salt, pepper, and spice to taste
Optional: ¼ cup dry oatmeal or Red River Cereal
Pre-heat oven to 350 º.
Put chicken onto greased or aluminum foil covered cookie sheet.
Apply barbeque sauce to each piece of chicken.
Mix pepper, salt, spices, and oatmeal together. Sprinkle mixture on top of barbeques sauce.
Place the cookie sheet into the oven and cook for 35 -45 minutes. Remove from oven and place chicken on a plate and serve.

Whole Roasted Chicken

Pre-heat oven to 425 º.
Clean and put breast side up in a casserole or roasting pan. Add ½ " to 1 "of water to the bottom of the pan. Sprinkle salt and pepper on top. Cover and place in oven and cook for 45 to 60 minutes (no pink left).
Remove from oven and pan, put slice up meat, wings, and legs on a plate and serve.

Fish - Cod, Halibut, or Sole

1 pound or 4 fillets of fish (thawed and drained)
2 medium zucchinis, sliced
½ cup carrots, shredded
½ small onion, cut into rings
Salt, pepper, seasoning to taste
1 tsp of garlic
½ cup shredded cheese (Monterey Jack, Mozzarella, or Cheddar)

Heat oven or grill.
On 18-inch square cookie sheet, cover with aluminum foil and place fish in the center. On top place carrots, zucchini, onions, seasoning, garlic, and cheese.
Fold and seal all edges (may need a second layer of foil). Place folded foil bundles on grill or in the oven.
Grill for about 10-14 minutes, or
Cook in oven 15 – 20 minutes or until fish flakes with a fork.
Open carefully steam may be hot!

Fish Pan Fried

Clean fish, remove skin and bones.
Using a frying pan melt butter and cook fish (sprinkle seasoning to taste)
Cook for 5 – 10 minutes, occasionally turn to other side. Remove and place on plate and serve.

Salmon

Whole Salmon, clean and sliced open belly
Mayonnaise
3-4 lemon slices
½ of Onion cut in rings
Salt, pepper, and spices to taste

In the belly, apply mayonnaise to both sides.
Place 3- 4 lemon slices beside each other.
On top of the lemon slices, place onions and sprinkle spices.
Apply mayonnaise to outside of both sides of the skin and place onto aluminum foil.
Fold and seal foil around the Salmon, place in the oven at 350° or grill on low heat.
Cook for 1 hour.
Open carefully and remove bones when eating.

Pork

THE DIFFERENCE BETWEEN HAM AND PORK?
Ham is particailly cooked when you buy it.

*You can buy different flavors of ham
(smoked, honey, etc.)

Oven - Roast   325°F

> Put into roasting pan, add 1 cup of water to pan.
> Spice as desired
> Cover with lid
> Place on lowest rack in oven, cook -depending on the size; 20 minutes/pound
> Every once in a while (10 minutes), check to make sure there is still a bit of water on the bottom of the pan.

Pan Fried

> Sliced Ham (Canadian Back Bacon is also great)
> Add a little water and cook the slices (flip over halfway through)
> Optional - Add onions, spices & mushrooms
>
> **Pork Chops** take approximately 20 minutes to cook. MUST NOT have any pink left in the center!

Barbequed

> Pork Chops (1 per/person) apply barbeque sauce.
> Cook on the barbeque (flip to cook both sides)

Pork Chops, Mashed Potatoes, Mushroom Soup & Peas

Make mashed potatoes (see recipe)
Pan fry the Pork Chops (1 per/person) in a bit of water (20 minutes – 10 each side)
Must not have any pink left in the center!
Optional - Add spices, onions & mushrooms (fry in pan with pork chops)
Add a can of mushroom soup, add a little more water to the pan if needed (should be like a sauce texture).
Add peas to pan and cook until tender.
Once all is cooked, place on plate and serve.

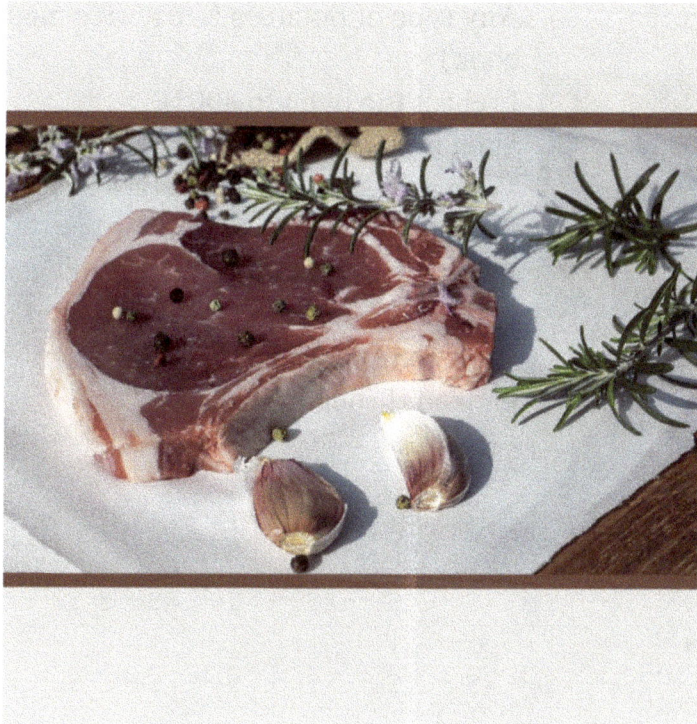

Potato

Baked Potato

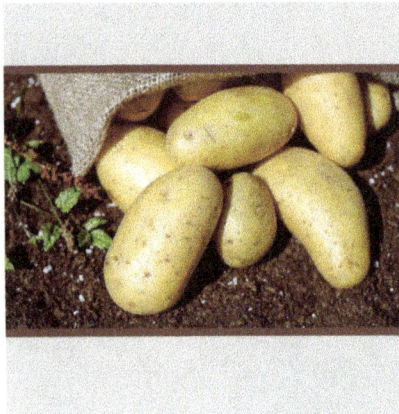

Any type of potatoes (small size might take less time to cook)

Preheat the oven to 400°F.

Under running water, scrub the potatoes clean.

With a fork, poke each potato in several places (so they do not explode).

Rub a little olive oil all over the potatoes.

Place directly on the middle rack of the oven.

Cook for 1 hour and 15 minutes, or until the potatoes are cooked through.

Hash Browns

Dice potato into small pieces
Melt butter in a fry pan on the stove
Add potatoes stir, and flip until tender
Add spices & onions

Mashed Potatoes

Any type of potatoes
Clean potatoes (can peel or not)
Cut up into cubes and place in pot of water (enough water to cover potatoes)
Boil until soft with a fork
Drain water
Add ¼ cup milk
2 tbsp butter
Mash with a potato masher or electric beater

Re-Fried Smashed Potatoes

Can use leftovers from last night <u>or</u>
Make mashed potatoes, then...
On the stove, melt butter in a fry pan
Add mashed potatoes
Flip as needed, should brown

Silver Dollars

Clean potatoes (can peel or not)
Slice into thin pieces. Should look like the size of a silver dollars or loonie.
On the stove, melt butter in a fry pan
Add potatoes stir & flip until tender
Add spices (& onions if desired)

Twice Baked Potatoes

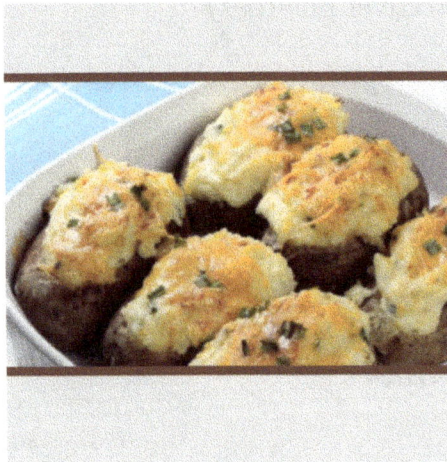

Preheat the oven to 400°F.

6 large russet potatoes
Olive oil

1st) Clean 6 russet large potatoes, under running water, scrub the potatoes clean.
With a fork, poke each potato in several places (so they do not explode).
Rub a little olive oil all over the potatoes.
Place directly on the middle rack of the oven.

➤ Cook at 400 º F   for 1 hour and 15 minutes, or until the potatoes are cooked through.
➤ Allow the potatoes to cool for 10 minutes
➤ Slice a third lengthwise off the top of each potato (creating a boat).
➤ Using a spoon to scoop out the cooked insides (forming a potato shell leaving about ¼ inch of potato on the skin) and place scooped out potato into a large mixing bowl.

2nd)
6 strips bacon
While the potatoes are cooking, cook the bacon in a frying pan until crisp (10 to 15 minutes). Drain on paper towels. Let cool. Crumble into small bits. Put to the side for later.

3rd)
¾ cup sour cream
¾ cup milk
3 Tbsp butter, softened
1 ½ Tbsp cream

Place the scooped-out potato insides, sour cream, milk, cream, and butter into a large bowl. Mash with a potato masher or an electric beater until desired consistency.

4th)
Topping - Cheddar cheese, bacon, and chives
1 ½ cup grated cheddar cheese
1/3 cup chopped green onion
¼ cup chopped fresh chives
½ tsp salt
½ tsp pepper

Mix a little of these toppings with the potatoes in step 3.

Reserve some of the toppings to sprinkle on the tops of the potatoes

5th)
Spoon mashed potatoes from the bowl into each potato shell.
Sprinkle with remainder of toppings.

6th)
To bake potatoes the second time
Re-heat the oven to 350°F. Place potatoes on a roasting pan or casserole dish and bake for another 15 minutes or until heated through.

Rice

Sushi

The rice is on the outside of the roll

How to cook rice

1. 2 cups medium short grain rice
2. Lots of water in a bowl. Put rice in and quickly wash it with your palm and drain.
3. Repeat until water is fairly clean
4. Drain water off.
5. Add 2 cups fresh water to rice
6. Soak the rice for 30 minutes or put in the electric rice maker
7. Cook the rice to a boil on high heat (lid on). Simmer for another 7 minutes.
8. Remove from heat.
9. Steam for 15 more minutes. (lid tight)

Sushi Vinegar

> 1 cup rice vinegar
> ½ cup sugar
> ½ tsp salt
> 1" x 3" kelp (seaweed) (keep in mixture for 30 minutes)
> Mix all sushi vinegar ingredients in a bowl, stir well.

Mix rice and sushi vinegar

Spread out rice, pour sushi vinegar over the rice and mix well. Not too much.

(½ cup sushi vinegar to 4 cups cooked rice)

Let rice cool, a fan will help

If need more time, cover with moist cloth.

California Rolls

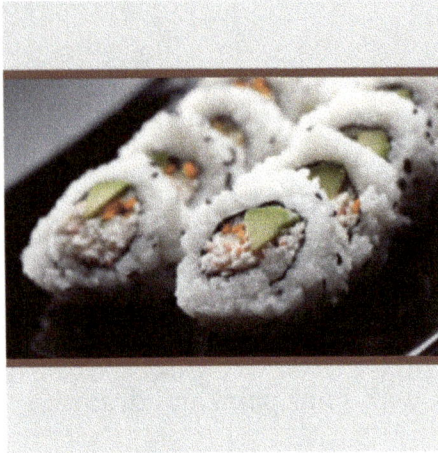

Makes 3 rolls

½ sliced avocados
2 sticks crab meat
Japanese Mayonnaise
1 ½ sheets of seaweed (Nori)
3 cups cooked rice
Sesame seeds or flying fish roe for topping

1. Completely cover a rolling mat with saran wrap. Cut a sheet of seaweed in half. On the rolling mat, lay 1 half cut seaweed sheet and spread 1 cup of sushi rice on it, covering the entire seaweed with rice.
2. Flip it over. Place the seaweed and rice at about 1 inch from bottom edge of rolling mat.
3. Put a little bit of Japanese Mayonnaise in center of seaweed.
4. Place 2 or three slices of avocado and crab (meat sticks) on the mayonnaise.
5. Put your two thumbs under the mat, pick up the bottom of the seaweed and tuck the part of the roll with the filling inside and roll the mat along with seaweed and rice.
6. Sprinkle sesame seeds on the roll and cut in 8 pieces
7. Serve with soy sauce, wasabi and or pickled ginger.
Optional; Replace crab with tuna, cooked chicken, or shrimp

Kappa Maki Roll

Rice is on the inside the of roll - Makes 3 rolls
3 strips English cucumber
1 ½ sheets seaweed
1 ½ cups cooked sushi rice

1. Cut a sheet of seaweed in half (shorter in length wise). Lay 1 half cut sheet on a rolling mat (shiny side down) and spread about ½ cup of cooked sushi rice thinly on the seaweed, leaving half inch of space at far side.
2. Lay 1 strip of cucumber in center of sushi rice.
3. Make sure seaweed is placed at bottom of the rolling mat.
4. Put your two thumbs under the mat, and roll the mat until the end touching the end of the sushi rice.
5. Lift the tip of the mat, and roll down 90 degree.
6. Place sushi roll, sealed part down so that seal does not open.
7. Cut into 6 pieces, serve with soy sauce, wasabi and or pickled ginger.

Rizza (Pizza)

350 º F 40 minutes   4-6 Servings
1 ½ cups of dry rice (Japanese sticky sushi rice is great) makes 3 cups for one rizza.
225 mls Pizza sauce per rizza
1 tablespoon oregano or pizza spice
Meat (choice of Chicken, shrimp, bacon, ham, hamburger, sausage, pepperoni, salami, or any other meat that you like on your pizza)
½ tsp butter
Choice of topping: Onion, green onions, peppers, pineapple, tomatoes, black olives, broccoli, spinach, or any other topping that you like on pizza.
½ cup of shredded mozzarella cheese
½ cup of grated Cheddar cheese (or any other kind you like on pizza: feta, parmesan)

Place a few Tbsp of the sauce and a ¼ tsp of spice into the water and cook the rice as the directions specify.
Grease or Butter the bottom of two pizza pans.
Place 3 cups of cooked rice onto pizza pan and spread and pat down to form the dough-look evenly on each pan. Spread remainder of pizza sauce onto Rizza and sprinkle some pizza spice over the rice.
Arrange meat evenly over Rizza. Add toppings evenly on Rizza. Sprinkle cheese on top.
Place into oven for 15 – 20 minutes or until cheese is melted. Slice into sections and serve on a plate. Tastes like pizza!

Main Dishes

Barley & Bacon Hotpot

1 ½ cups pearl barley
½ lb bacon, cut up
2 Tbsp butter
2 large onion, chopped
1 ½ cups carrots, thinly diced
1 cup celery, chopped
2 cups mushroom, thinly chopped
3 cups chicken broth
4 Tbsp parsley, chopped
Salt & pepper to taste

Preheat oven to 350°. Melt butter in Dutch oven or large roasting pan. Add bacon & onions, cook gently for 5 minutes (until the onions are soft & slightly cooked). Stir in carrots, celery, mushrooms, and pear barly. Then pour in the broth and bring to a boil. Add parsley, salt, and pepper. Cover, for one hour or until barley is soft and nearly all liquid is absorbed. Serve hot.

Barbequed Pork & Bean Bake

Step 1)
1 lb white beans (soaked in water over night)
Boil soaked beans until soft (about 2 hours)
Drain off (reserving 3 cups of liquid). Set aside.

Step 2)
Marinade 1 lb uncooked pork (cubed) in 2 tsp liquid smoke for about 10 minutes.

Step 3)
1 large onion, diced
½ cup celery, chopped

Step 4)
Add pork, celery, onions to beans (use large roasting pan)
Stir.

Step 5) Add
1 cup brown sugar
1 Tbsp white vinegar
1 Tbsp dry mustard
2 cups ketchup
½ cups molasses
¼ cup Tony Romas hickory BBQ sauce
½ tsp salt

Step 6) Stir well. Bake at 325° F for 2 ½ - 3 hours.

Chili

½ pound ground hamburger

¼ to ½ onion

3 stalks celery chopped

Salt & Pepper to taste

1-2 cans of brown beans

1 can kidney beans

1 Tbsp white vinegar

1 Tbsp brown sugar

Optional – corn, or any other vegetable

Brown hamburger & add onions and celery stir 2 minutes. Add all remaining ingredients, simmer for 1 – 2 hours.

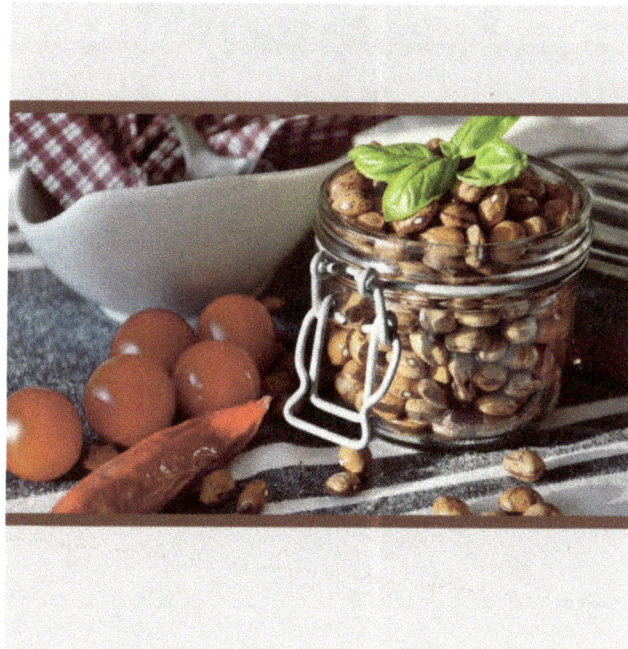

Steamed Vegetables

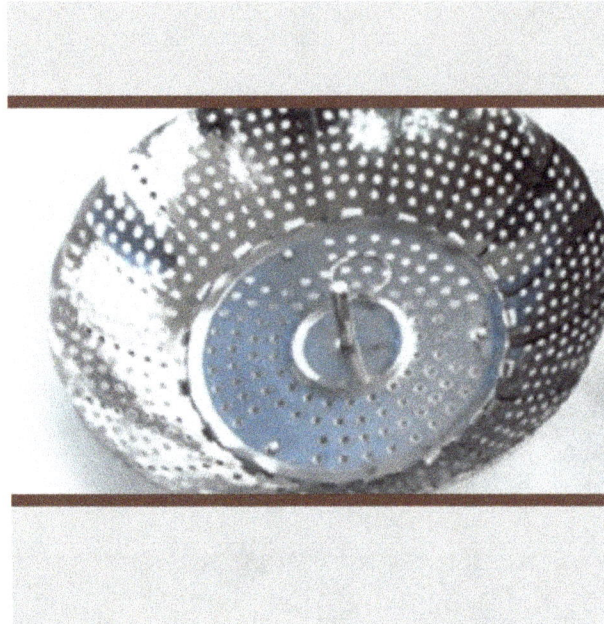

Your choice of vegetables: broccoli, cauliflower, carrots, peas, etc.

Place vegetables in a steaming machine, double boiler, or this type of vegetable steamer.
- About 1 inch of water is filled in the pot.
- Cleaned and chopped vegetables are placed in steamer.
- Steamer is place into the water
- Pot is on the stove medium high temperature.

Zucchini Lasagna

Serves 6   400 °F   45 -55 minutes
1-pound hamburger
1 slice bacon, cut up
1 can tomato sauce or ½ jar of your favourite spaghetti sauce
Pinch of salt, pepper, oregano, Italian spice & garlic powder
1 small onion
1 cup fresh spinach
¼ cup water
4 large zucchinis, thinly sliced length wise
½ red pepper, cleaned and diced
500 mls of cottage cheese
2 cups cheddar or mozzarella cheese

On stove top in large pot brown hamburger, salt and pepper, bacon, onions, sauce, water, and spinach.
In large glass 9 x 11 casserole dish layer
- Zucchini covering bottom evenly
- ½ of cooked hamburger mix
- Zucchini layer
- Cottage cheese layer
- Other ½ of cooked hamburger mix
- Sprinkle with cheese on top

Bake in oven

Add a salad to any meal!

Desserts

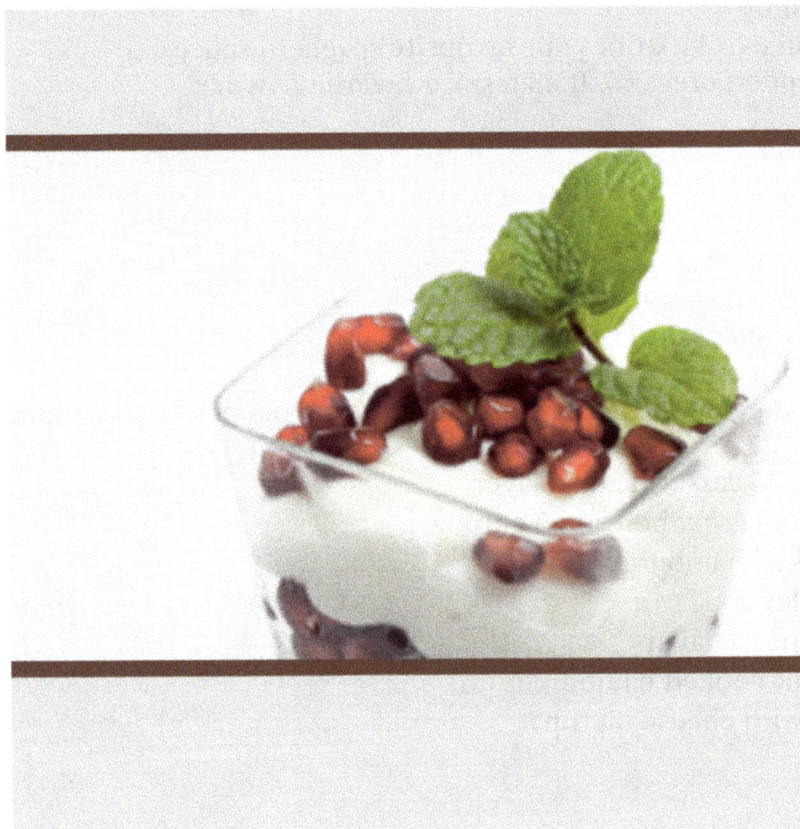

Almond Crust Recipe

2 cups Almond flour
If want chocolate – add 2- 4 Tbsp cocoa powder
½ cup sugar
1 tsp Cinnamon
Pinch of Salt
½ cup butter

- ➢ Lightly toast almond flour in a dry skillet or pan over medium heat, until fully golden and fragrant (2-4 minutes). This is very important taste-wise, so do not skip!
- ➢ Transfer toasted almond flour to a small bowl (or go straight for the serving glass), and mix in sweetener, cinnamon, and salt. Add in butter, mix until thoroughly combined. Press into the pie dish
- ➢ NOTE: you can alternatively use this crust for a baked pie or tart too. The crust itself (i.e. blind-baked) will cook in about 10-18 minutes at 350°F/180°C (depending on size).or serving glass and refrigerate while you make the filling.

Baked Apple

450° F - 60 Minutes, Per person
1 Apple (your choice of type)
¼ tsp Cinnamon
1 tsp Brown Sugar
½ tsp Butter
1/8 cup Oatmeal

OR

½ Apple (your choice of type)
½ Banana
4 Strawberries
10 Blueberries
½ tsp Cinnamon
2 tsp Brown Sugar
1 tsp Butter
¼ cup Oatmeal

Cut the apple(s) in quarters and remove the core. *Peeling is optional.*
Cut remaining apple into bit size pieces and place into a casserole dish. Add cinnamon, brown sugar, oatmeal, and butter. Place into oven and cook.
Remove from oven and put into a bowl and eat. *Optional, can add whip topping or cream on top.*

Carmel Fruit Dip

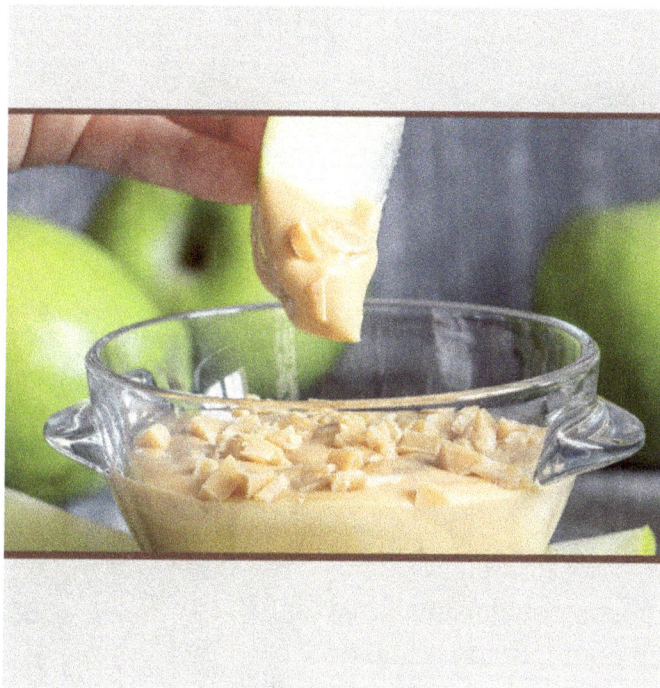

1 cup Cream Cheese
1/3 cup Brown Sugar
¼ tsp vanilla extract
½ tsp of Carmel extract (optional)

Mix well and chill
Cut up apples, melons, or strawberries. Dip and eat.

Chilled Chocolate Slice

2 eggs slightly beaten
1 ½ cups icing sugar
2 squares melted chocolate
1 tsp vanilla
> ➤ Mix these ingredients well, then add.
½ lb of mini marshmallows
1 cup chopped walnuts
1 cup shredded coconut (optional)
Blend well, then pour into buttered pan & chill

Optional – Chocolate Icing Sugar
½ cup butter, melted
2/3 cup unsweetened cocoa powder
3 cups powdered sugar
1/3 cup milk
1 tsp vanilla extract
Stir melted butter and cocoa powder in a bowl until evenly mixed. Add confectioners' sugar and milk; beat until smooth and easily spread. Stir in vanilla extract.

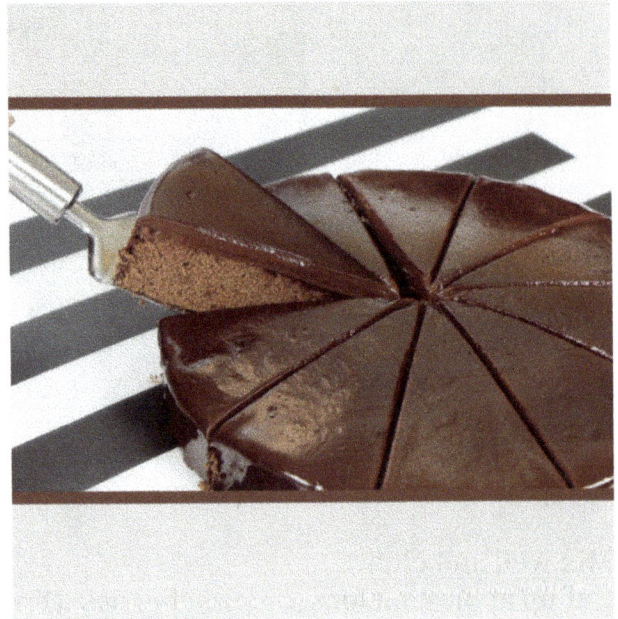

Cheesecake

Step 1)
1500-gram Philadelphia cream cheese (room temperature)
- ➤ Take off less than a ¼ of the cream cheese block
- ➤ Slice into ½" pieces, add to blender
- ➤ Mix 20 seconds (looks like soft butter)

Step 2)
Flavour Choices
Choice #1
> 1 small can of pineapple
> ¼ tsp coconut extract (½ cap)
> 1 tsp vanilla extract (2 caps full)

Choice #2
> 1 small can of pineapple
> 1 ½ oz Kahlua
> 1 tsp vanilla extract (2 caps full)

Choice #3
> 8 oz melted chocolate

Choice #4
> 3 mars or similar kind of chocolate
> bars

Choice #5
> ½ cup coffee & 4 oz of chocolate,
> Kahlua, or Baileys

Choice #6
> 1 cup of diced fruit

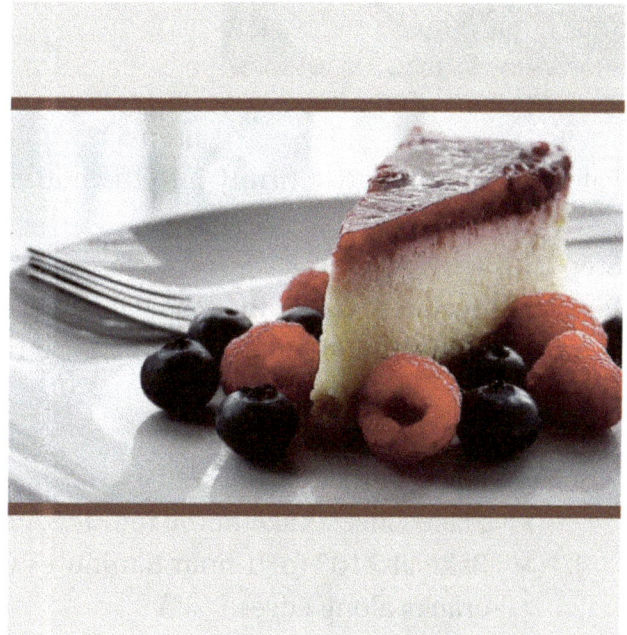

Add to the cream cheese and flavor

Step 3)

Add to the cream cheese and flavor (mix a little at a time)
1½ cups whipping cream
¾ cup of sugar
5 slightly beaten large eggs

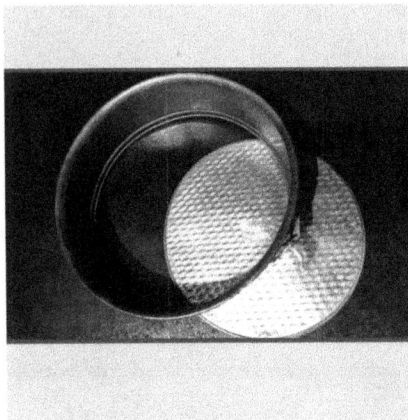

Step 4)
Put pan together and butter (bottom & sides)
I use a bit of saran wrap to hold the butter while I smear it on the surfaces.

Step 5)
Pat down almond crust firmly into the buttered pan (see recipe).

Step 6)
Pour cream cheese batter into the pan (over top of the almond crust)
➢ Spin the pan fast & carefully until there is lots of bubbles at the top

Step 7)
➢ Place ½ inch of water in a broiling pan on the bottom shelf of the oven.
➢ Place Cheesecake in the middle of the oven,
➢ Bake at 310° for 1 hour 5 minutes (watch for last five minutes). Look for tiny cracks along edges (¼")
Set 8 hours at room temperature (off the countertop – on stand/rack).
Cool in fridge 16 hours (Keeps for two weeks).
Add fruit and whip cream, serve

Chocolate

Yep, chocolate is angelic!

Chocolate Unbaked Oatmeal Cookies

2 cups sugar
½ cup butter
½ cup milk
3 cups oatmeal
½ cup cocoa
1 tsp vanilla extract
½ tsp of salt
Boil together sugar, butter, milk, salt and coco for five minutes. Add Oatmeal, coconut. Stir all together. Remove from heat. Take large spoonful's (cookie size) and drop onto paraffin covered cookie sheet, will have interesting shapes. Let cool to room temperature and serve.

Fruit Granita

4 servings
Ice cream or sherbet replacement
Granita is grainy textured icy mixture of water, sugar and flavouring frozen in a pan in the freezer. The goal when making granita is to create coarse granular crystals or flakes of ice.

1 cup water
2/3 cups white sugar
2 cups of fresh or frozen strawberries, pureed. (raspberrics or 6 peaches)
Optional: Sweetened whipped cream

Hull and puree the strawberries in a food processor.
Choose a large, shallow pan (8 x 12 x 2-inches) that allows the mixture to spread out.
While you are assembling the recipe, place the empty pan and your stirring fork in the freezer to chill. Also chill the glasses you will be using to serve the granita in later.

Making syrup; cook water and sugar until sugar is dissolved and an additional 3 – 4 minutes longer. Add to strawberries, chill thoroughly. Once chilled put into shallow pan and freeze 3 to 4 hours, using a fork stirring every 30 minutes break up the frozen parts near the edges into smaller chunks, scraping mixture into fine particles and rake them toward the center. Continue to freeze and break up ice crystals until completely frozen, about 3 to 4 hours.

(Can also be made according to ice cream maker's instructions).

Scoops and serve in chilled dessert dish, goblet, wine glass or in a center of half honeydew melon. Top with a spoonful of whipped cream. Garnish with berries, lemon zest, or a sprig fresh mint leaf.

Lemon Granita

4-5 large lemons
2 cups water
1 cup sugar

Cut all the lemons in half and squeeze them to get juice.
In a medium saucepan, combine the water and sugar. Bring to a boil.
Lower heat to simmer, add the lemon juice, and stir to dissolve the sugar.
Transfer the mixture to a shallow pan and place in the freezer.
Freeze according to the instructions for freezing granita above.

Cut long strips of lemon rind from 2 of the lemons
Add the lemon peel strips as garnish.

Fruit,

Any type (optional - add whipped cream).

Fruit Salad

1 orange
½ apple
½ pear
½ banana
½ nectarine
10 grapes halved
Sprinkle of coconut
Optional: Sweetened whipped cream

Combine all together. Serve in dessert dish and top with a spoonful of whipped cream.

Pumpkin Pie

4 eggs
1 can 796 ml E.D Smith PURE 100% Pumpkin
2 cups brown sugar
2 tsp ground cinnamon
1 tsp ground nutmeg
1 tsp ground ginger
½ tsp salt
1 can evaporated milk

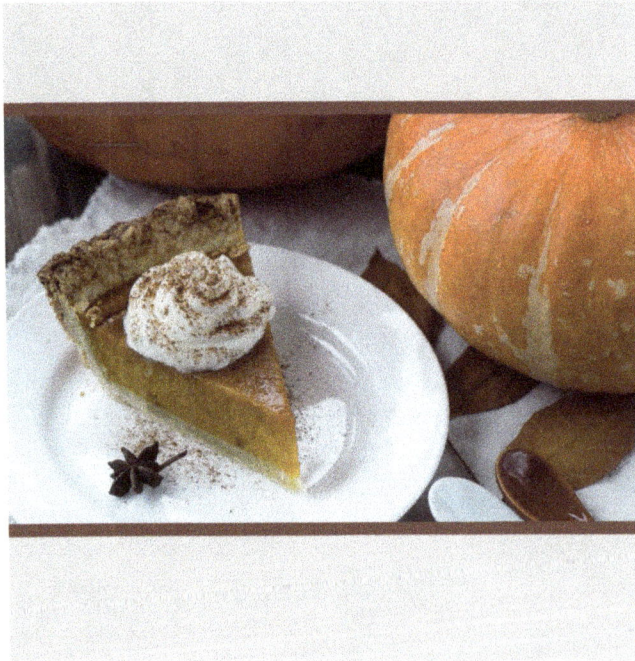

Beat eggs, add all ingredients (except milk), mix.
Blend in milk.
Choice – no crust or have almond crust bottom. Pour filling into pie plate.
Bake at 425° 15 minutes, reduce oven temperature to 350° and continue baking 30 -35 minutes, longer or until toothpick inserted in center comes out clean.
Cool.

Vanilla Yogurt

With any type of fruit topping.

Vanilla Ice Cream

With any type of fruit topping or sprinkle dried Cocoa over top.

Vanilla Ice Cream Dessert

1 cup boiling water
1 red jello (dissolve in water)
1 can fruit cocktail (drain and keep juice)
½ cup of the drained fruit juice
1 brick (500ml) vanilla ice cream (chilled not frozen)

Combine all together and chill.

5 Minute Fudge

2/3 cup carnation evaporated milk

1 2/3 cups white sugar

¼ tsp salt

> ➤ In saucepan, over medium heat, bring to boil. Stirring constantly, cook 5 minutes.
> ➤ Remove from heat

Add

1½ cup (16) diced marshmallows

1½ cups chocolate chips

1 tsp vanilla

½ cup chopped walnuts

Stir 1-2 minutes until marshmallows melt. Pour into butterde 9" square pan. Chill.

Drinks

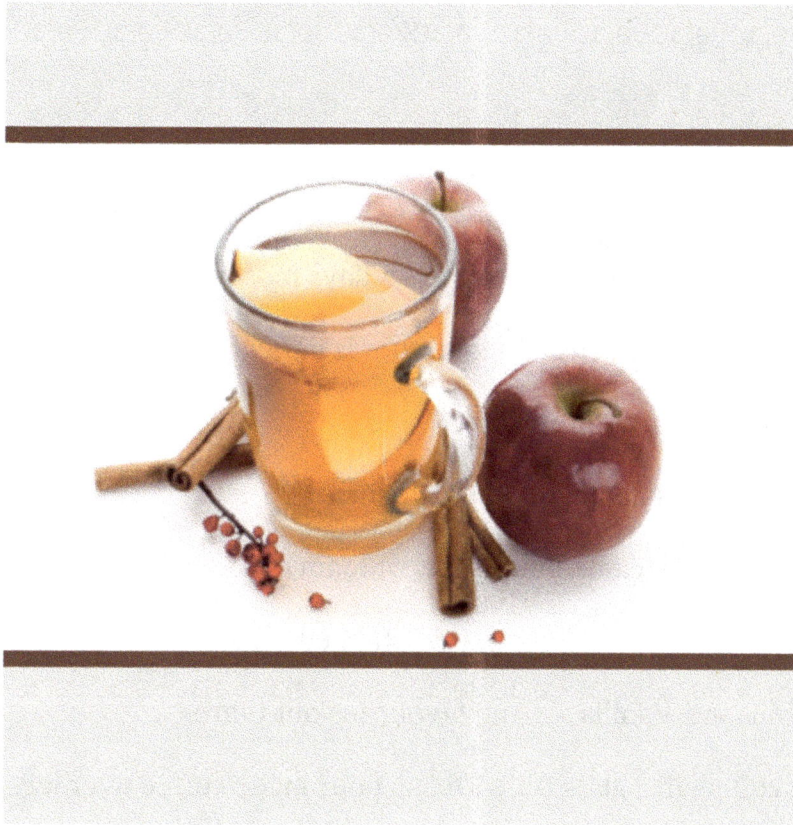

Chai Latte

Heat a cup of milk in the microwave or steam. Add tea bags -seep or three Tbsp of Chai tea powder.
Stir and drink

Coffee

(cream and sugar are okay but watch out for weight gain)
- Coffee - Traditional
  - Fine drip or percolated
  - Use to be the Robusta plant, now- a-days most use the Arabica plant
- Espresso
  - Very Strong coffee (usually one shot is enough, 2 oz)
- Americano
  - Espresso with hot water
- Latte
  - Espresso with steamed milk (no foam)
- Cappuccino
  - Espresso with steamed milk (lots of foam)
- Mocha
  - Latte with a shot of Chocolate & whipped cream
- Flavoured
  - Hazelnut and Vanilla are the favourites out there.
- Ice Coffee
  - Make coffee; in a glass fill with ice, pour made coffee over ice.

Fruit Juice

Fruit of any kind (Cranberry / Pineapple mixed is great or Cranberry /Orange)
Vegetable Juice
>Using juicer; juice any vegetables (I like to drain the foam off first with a strainer and then drink).

Hot Chocolate

1 cup hot milk
1 tablespoon Cocoa
½ to 1 tablespoon sugar
Pinch ground cinnamon
>Combine and stir.
>>Optional; top with whip cream and sprinkle with cinnamon

Iced Tea

(Snapple brand is one of the healthiest)
Sun Brewed (Fun to try)
>Fill a container with 4 cups of cold water. Place 6 bags or 6 tsps of your favourite tea and cover lightly. Place in direct sunlight for 2 to 4 hours (depending on desired strength). Remove bags or strain and serve over ice.
>>Optional: add sugar to taste
Cold Water Method

Fill a container with 4 cups of cold water. Place 6 bags or 6 tsp of tea and cover lightly. Place in the refrigerator for 8 hours. Remove bags or strain and serve over ice.

Optional: add sugar to taste

Lemonade

Serves 6

    1 cup sugar (less if desired)
    1 cup water, to dissolve

    1 cup lemon juice (4-6 lemons)
    3 to 4 cups cold water (to dilute)

In a pot on the stove add the sugar and water, dissolve completely.

While the sugar is dissolving, you can use a juicer to extract the juice from the 4 to 6 lemons (enough for one cup of juice) or a handheld plastic juicer.

In a pitcher combine the 3 to 4 cups of cold water (desired strength), the lemon juice and sugar water. Stir. Refrigerate 30 to 40 minutes.

You can change the sweetness by adding a little more lemon juice or water to it.

Serve with ice and sliced lemons.

London Fog Tea

Heat a cup of milk in the microwave or steam.
Add 1 Earl Gray tea bag -seep
Add 1 tsp of Vanilla
Stir and drink

Milk

Cow's milk (skim to 2% - cream is okay, but fattening)
Rice
Soy

Smoothie

½ cup Yogurt (vanilla)
½ cup Juice (apple, orange, etc.) or Water (or as needed) or Milk
½ cup Ice
1 cup Fruit (fresh or frozen)
½ banana (optional)
½ tsp flax seeds or oil (optional)
Combine all ingredients in a blender. Cover and turn on until smooth. Pour into glass and drink.

Tea of any kind

Seep in a cup of hot water (can use tea bags or tea infuser)

Water

Optional; add lemon to taste
Hot, warm, or cold

Wheat Grass

It provides chlorophyll, amino acids, minerals, vitamins, and enzymes
You will need a special wheat grass blender.
Cut the desired amount of Wheat Grass, put into blender and grind.
Drink alone or in mixed fruit or vegetable drinks

Bonus

**Other interesting
ways you
can change up the
Angelic Foods**

Introduction to Ayurvedic Diet

What's your Dosha? Are you more of a Vata, Piita or Kapha?

VATA

Skin: Dry, thin, fine-pored & delicate skin which is prone to wrinkles & excessive dryness.   May become rough & flaky.
Hair: Thin, dark, sometimes frizzy or course & tends to be dry
Lips: thin, often dry & cracked
Body: Thin & doesn't gain weight easily
Sleep: Difficulty falling asleep & often interrupted
Temperament: Enthusiastic & vivacious by nature. Tends to be nervous.
Mind: Alert, active, imaginative, sometimes restless
Endurance: Low, easily exhausted
Memory: Quick but also forgets quickly

PITTA

Skin: Reddish or freckled complexion. Sensitive to sunlight.
Hair: Normal to fine. Thin, reddish or light. Tends to grey prematurely.
Lips: Medium-sized, red or pink.
Body: Medium frame, well built.
Sleep: Sound. Requires medium amount of sleep.
Temperament: Motivated. Easily irritated or angered. Tends to be critical.
Mind: Energetic, intelligent, assertive & organized.
Endurance: Moderate, but not focused.
Memory: Sharp & clear.

KAPHA

Skin: Thick, moist, pale complexion.
Hair: Normal to oily. Thick, wavy, dark & shiny.
Lips: Thick, pale.
Body: Large frame. Weight is easy to gain & hard to lose. Tends to be overweight.
Sleep: Sound, long & heavy. Needs at least 8 hours sleep.
Temperament: Sympathetic, courageous, forgiving, loving.
Mind: Calm & content. Easily depressed.
Endurance: High, good stamina. Steady level of energy.
Memory: Slow, unflinching & steady.

The six flavors:

Sweet: grains, milk, rice, sugar & honey
Sour: vinegar, yogurt, cheese & lemons
Salty: salt & soy sauce
Bitter: bitter greens, tonic water, lemon rind, spinach & rhubarb
Pungent: cayenne, chili peppers, onions, garlic, ginger & radishes
Astringent: beans, lentils, cabbage, broccoli, apples & pomegranates

These flavors help determine whether a food is *heating* or *cooling*. Generally, sour, salty and pungent tastes are heating, whereas sweet, bitter and astringent are cooling.
The six Qualities: which come in pairs, are:

Heavy or Light - wheat is heavy, barley is light; beef is heavy, chicken is light; cheese is heavy, skim milk is light
Oily or Dry - milk is oily, honey is dry; soybeans are oily, lentils are dry; coconut is oily, cabbage is dry
Hot or Cold (heats or cools the body) - pepper is hot, mint is cold; honey is hot, sugar is cold; eggs are hot, milk is cold

Foods that you would eat in your Doshas type are:

VATA:

Balances	**Aggravates**
Sweet	Pungent
Sour	Bitter
Salty	Astringent
Heavy	Light
Oily	Dry
Hot	Cold
Cooked vegetables	Raw vegetables
Stewed fruits	Dried fruits
Sweet, well ripened fruit	Unripe fruit
Oats, rice, wheat	Barley, buckwheat, corn, dry oats, millet, rye
All dairy	
Chicken, turkey, seafood (all in small amounts)	Red meat
Chickpeas, mung beans, Pink lentils, tofu	All beans except noted

All oils are acceptable.
All sweeteners are acceptable.
All nuts & seeds are acceptable in small amounts.
Almost all herbs & spices in moderation, with emphasis on sweet &/or heating herbs & spices.
No spice should be used in large quantities. Minimize all bitter & astringent herbs & spices.

PITTA:

Balances	Aggravates
Sweet	Pungent
Bitter	Sour
Astringent	Salty
Cold	Hot
Heavy	Light
Dry	Oily
Raw vegetables in summer	
Sweet & ripe fruit	Avoid sour & unripe fruit
Barley, oats, wheat, white rice	Brown rice, corn, millet, rye
Butter, egg whites, ghee	Buttermilk, cheese, egg yolks
Ice cream, milk	Sour cream, yogurt
Chicken, turkey, shrimp	Red meat & seafood in general
(all in small amounts)	
Chickpeas, mung beans,	Lentils
Tofu & other soybean products	
Coconut, olive, soy & sunflowers oils	Almond, corn, safflower, sesame oils

All sweeteners are acceptable, except honey & molasses

Avoid all nuts & seeds except coconut, pumpkin & sunflower seeds.

Spices are generally avoided as they are too heating, but some sweet, bitter, & astringent ones are good in small amounts.

KAPHA:

Balances	Aggravates
Pungent	Sweet
Bitter	Sour
Astringent	Salty
Light	Heavy
Dry	Oily
Hot	Cold
All vegetables	Sweet & juicy vegetables
Dried fruits	Sweet, sour, or very juicy fruits
Barley, buckwheat, corn, millet, rye	Oats, rice, wheat
	Avoid hot cereals & streamed grains
Skim milk	Avoid all dairy except for small amounts of whole milk & eggs
Chicken, turkey, shrimp (all in small amounts)	red meat & seafood in general
All legumes, except as noted	Kidney beans & tofu
Almond, corn, safflower, sunflower Oils (all in small amounts)	All oils except as noted
Avoid all sweeteners, except raw, unheated honey.	
Avoid al nuts & seeds except for sunflower & pumpkin seeds.	
All herbs & spices	Salt

The Five Element Diet

Great to try in the different seasons of the year or if you have been to a Chinese doctor and they told you what element you are. Then you would eat mostly from that group of foods

Five energies of foods – Cold, hot, warm, cool, and neutral
Light flavors promote urination – diuretics
> Cucumber
> Job's tears

Wood Element – Spring
Sour Flavors – lemon, lime, pickles, sauerkraut, crab apple, plum, peach
Chicken, mandarin, orange, pineapple, raspberry, strawberry
liver, mango, tomato, vinegar, avocado, olive, zucchini, lettuce, peas, loquat
parsley, litchi, string beans, kumquat, broccoli, grapefruit, wheat, grape
apple, apricot

Fire Element – Summer
Bitter flavors – Alfalfa, bitter melon, romaine lettuce, rye
Tomato, vinegar, raspberry wine, strawberry, apricot, red beans, brussels sprouts
corn, quinoa, sea grass, asparagus, bitter gourd, wild cucumber, celery, cherry seeds, coffee,
grapefruit peel, kohlrabi, lettuce, radish leaf, animals' gallbladder

Earth Element –Late Summer
Sweet flavors – Honey Molasses, whole sugar, beef, pork, celery, chicken, duck, eel,
mutton, pork, Apple, Cherry, Coconut, carrots, brown sugar, banana, barley, date, beetroot,
black sesame seeds, black soybean, Chinese cabbage, fig, chestnut, eggs, cinnamon, fresh
white clams, carrot, coffee, common button mushroom, corn, crab apple, cucumber,
squash, red and black date, eggplant, ginseng, grape, sweet potato, grapefruit, guava, honey,
kidney beans, kohlrabi, kumquat, yam, lettuce, licorice, litchi, olive, oyster, papaya, peach,
peanuts, watermelon, milk, malt, mandarin, orange, mango, pineapple, plum, potato,
pumpkin, radish, raspberry, rice bran, rice

Metal Element – Autumn
Pungent Flavors – Cayenne, black pepper, hot green and red peppers, fresh ginger
Castor beans, radish, spearmint, star anise, sweet basil, taro, rice bran, cherry seeds, tobacco, wine, soybeans, chives, navy beans, nutmeg, cauliflower, cinnamon bark, garlic, Chinese parsley, soybean oil, green onion, cottonseed, rosemary, turnip, dill seed, leaf mustard
Peach, fennel, leek, marjoram, pear, grapefruit peel, peppermint, kohlrabi, kumquat
Slightly Pungent – Asparagus, caraway

Water Element – Winter
Salty Flavors –
Salt, seaweed, soy sauce, miso, kelp, pork, abalone, barley, cranberry, blueberry, blackberry, chive seeds, clams, oysters, human's milk, duck, saffron, sesame oil, shitake mushroom, shrimp, soybean oil, spearmint, spinach, squash, star anise, strawberry, string bean, sugar cane, sunflower seed, sweet rice, sword bean, tomato, walnut, water chestnut, wheat, white sugar, wine, yellow soybean

Meridian Body & Eating Clock

Depending on what time of the day it is, will determine which meridian/organ is working or asleep. Each meridian has a 2-hour time frame (am – pm) and has different requirements.

Meridian Eating Clock

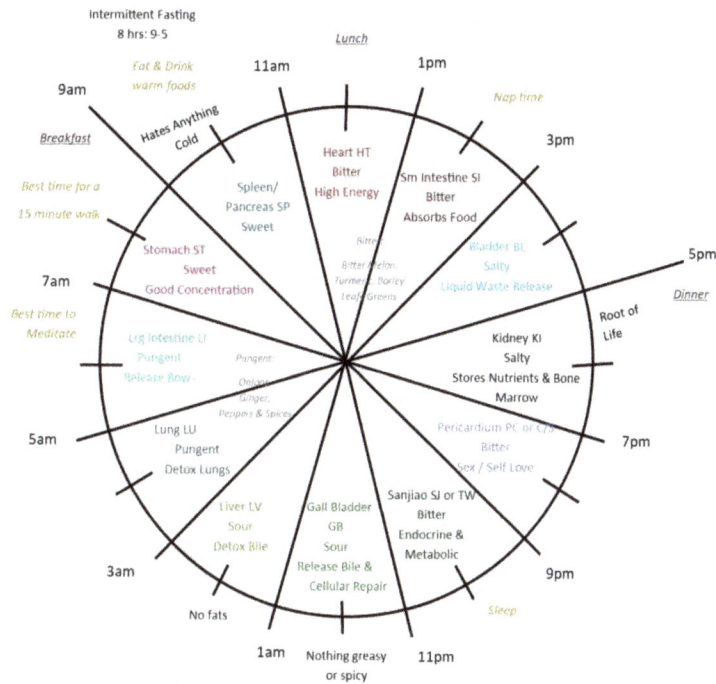

Meridian Eating Clock diagram showing:

- **Intermittent Fasting** 8 hrs: 9-5 — *Eat & Drink warm foods*
- **9am** — Spleen/Pancreas SP, Sweet — *Hates Anything Cold*
- **Breakfast** — *Best time for a 15 minute walk*
- **11am** — Heart HT, Bitter, High Energy
- **Lunch** — *Bitter, Bitter Melon, Turmeric, Barley, Leafy Greens*
- **1pm** — Sm Intestine SI, Bitter, Absorbs Food — *Nap time*
- **3pm** — Bladder BL, Salty, Liquid Waste Release
- **5pm** — Kidney KI, Salty, Stores Nutrients & Bone Marrow — Root of Life
- **Dinner**
- **7pm** — Pericardium PC or CX, Bitter, Sex / Self Love
- **7am** — Stomach ST, Sweet, Good Concentration — *Best time to Meditate*
- **9pm** — Sanjiao SJ or TW, Bitter, Endocrine & Metabolic
- **5am** — Lung LU, Pungent, Detox Lungs — Lrg Intestine LI, Pungent, Release Bowels
- *Pungent, Onion, Ginger, Peppers & Spices*
- **11pm** — Gall Bladder GB, Sour, Release Bile & Cellular Repair — *Sleep*
- **3am** — Liver LV, Sour, Detox Bile
- **1am** — *Nothing greasy or spicy*
- **No fats**

CONSTANCE SANTEGO.CA

Shift happens... Create magic!

Source points and zipping up a meridian can balance by weakening or strengthen the meridian/organ.

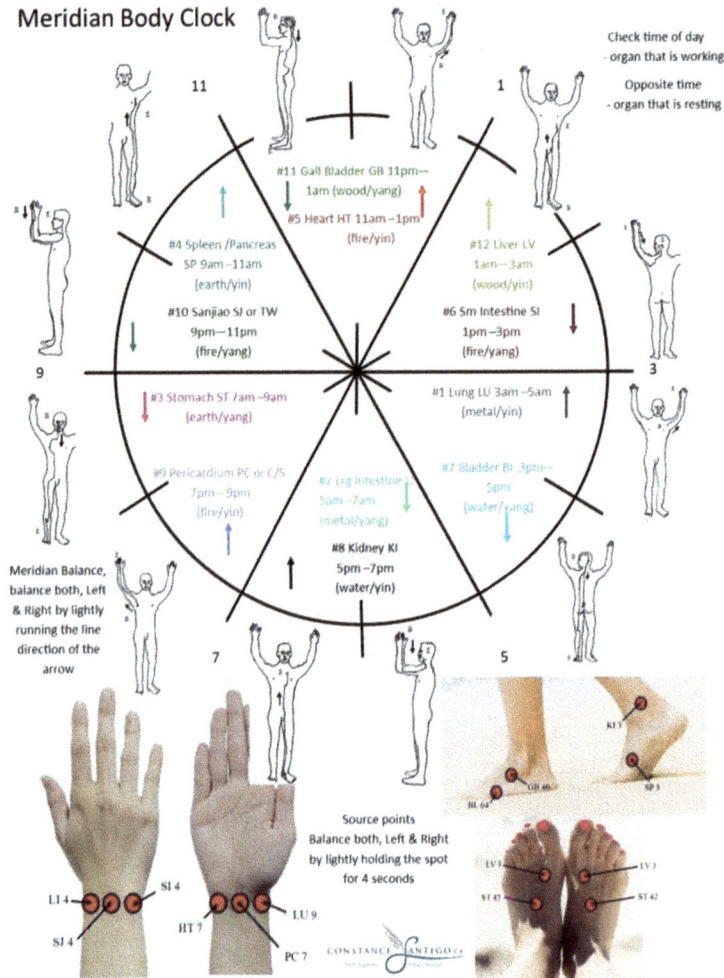

Meridian Body Clock

Check time of day
- organ that is working

Opposite time
- organ that is resting

#11 Gall Bladder GB 11pm—1am (wood/yang)

#5 Heart HT 11am—1pm (fire/yin)

#4 Spleen /Pancreas SP 9am—11am (earth/yin)

#12 Liver LV 1am—3am (wood/yin)

#10 Sanjiao SJ or TW 9pm—11pm (fire/yang)

#6 Sm Intestine SI 1pm—3pm (fire/yang)

#3 Stomach ST 7am—9am (earth/yang)

#1 Lung LU 3am—5am (metal/yin)

#9 Pericardium PC or C/S 7pm—9pm (fire/yin)

#2 Lrg Intestine 5am—7am (metal/yang)

#7 Bladder Bl 3pm—5pm (water/yang)

#8 Kidney KI 5pm—7pm (water/yin)

Meridian Balance, balance both, Left & Right by lightly running the line direction of the arrow

Source points
Balance both, Left & Right by lightly holding the spot for 4 seconds

LI 4   SI 4
SJ 4   HT 7   LU 9
        PC 7

KI 3   GB 40   SP 3
Bl. 64

LV 1   LV 3
ST 43   ST 42

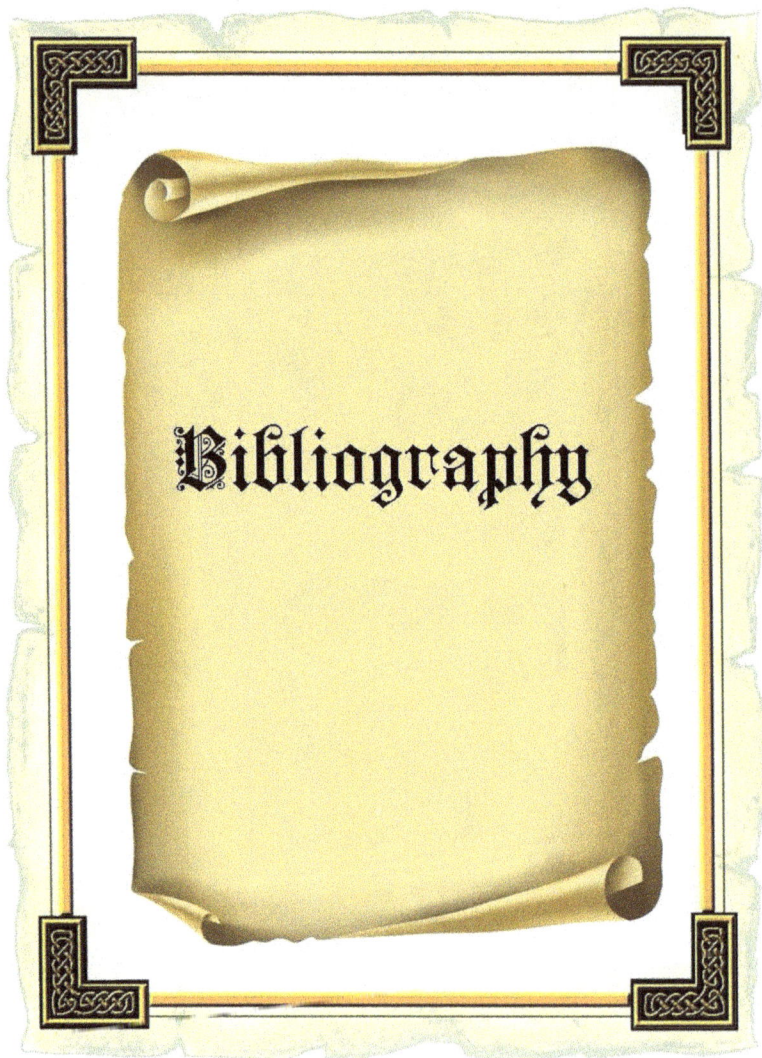

Bibliography

I received ideas of book design and some types of menu plans from these places:

My Grandmother's, Mom's and other family member's recipes

The parents of my son's grade three class (the kids made a recipe book)

Hamlyn
1977 The Best of Cooking, Hamlyn publishing group

Istockphotos.com

J.R Watkins Fine Spices

Land O'Lakes Test Kitchens & Robin Krause
1994 Treasury of Country Heritage Meals and Menus, Tormont Publications

Mike Snyder with Nancy Faass
2010 The Everything Raw Food Recipe Book, F & W Media

Nathan Hyam
2004-2010 Salad Dressing 101, Whitecap books

Prescription for Nutritional Healing Phyllis A Balch,

Websites:

https://www.disabled-world.com/medical/supplements/vitamins/

http://www.cryst.bbk.ac.uk/education/AminoAcid/the_twenty.html

https://cookieandkate.com/how-to-make-tzatziki/

https://thewanderlustkitchen.com/authentic-greek-tzatziki/

https://www.gnom-gnom.com/paleo-keto-graham-cracker-pie-crust/

https://www.allrecipes.com/recipe/234702/quick-almond-flour-pancakes/

https://www.delish.com/cooking/recipe-ideas/recipes/a56226/cauliflower-garlic-bread-recipe/

Message From The Author

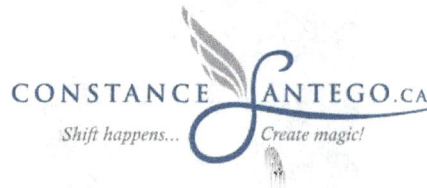

CONSTANCE ANTEGO.CA

Shift happens...   *Create magic!*

Developing your Intuitive Energy takes time and patience. These Angelic foods are what gave me the title of 'Grand' Reiki Master. I did the 42-Day cleanse seven times in a row. It was to teach me self-discipline at the same time as cleansing my Body, Mind, and Soul.

Take the ideas I give you and tweak them if need be. You are your own master and have the power within you to do great things in this lifetime.

From my heart to yours, enjoy!

Constance

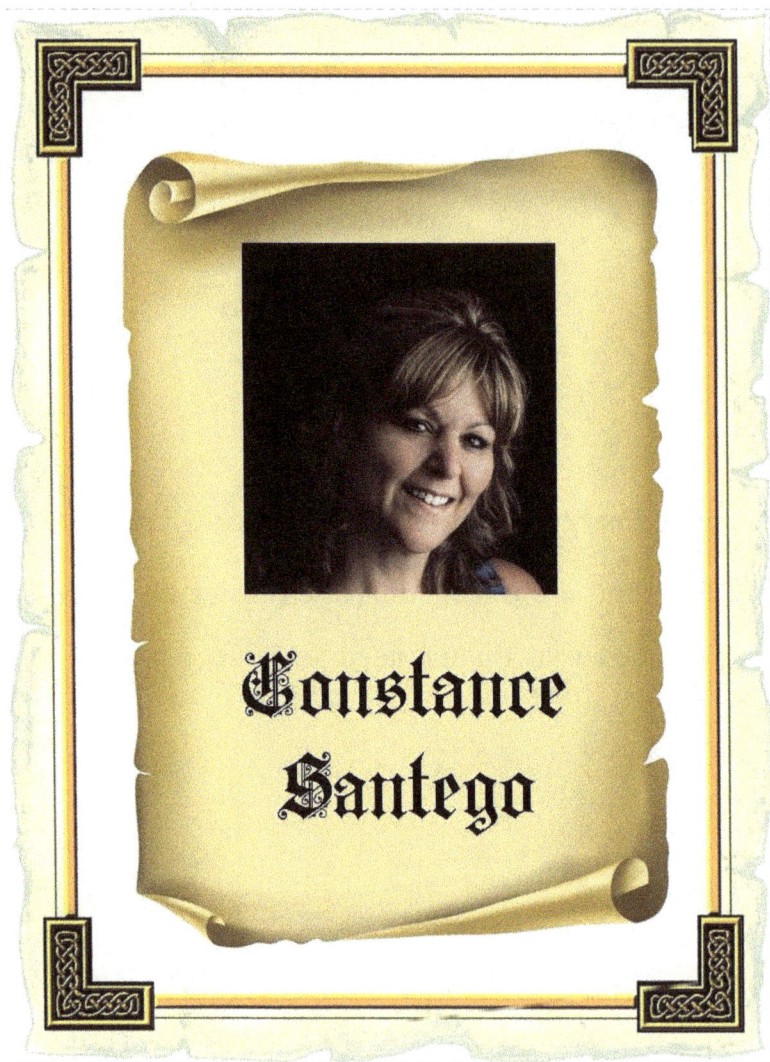

Constance
Santego

Shift happens...Create magic!
Dream BIGGER!

Constance Santego is an Author, Grand Reiki Master, Master Educator and Healer of the Holistic and Spiritual Arts. She is known for bridging the body, mind, and soul consciousness to create your dreams into reality.

Constance's background is in business, owning her first company at the age of twenty-seven until her back went out and she had to sell. Learning how to heal herself holistically, she gained many, many certificates and diplomas in spirituality and natural healing from amazing schools around the world.

In 1999, she opened a school that became accredited in the holistic arts and ran that until 2012 teaching students from all over the world how to heal themselves and others.

The art of healing seems to open a gate to quantum energy, where magic seems to be taking place. But it must be a science since if I can teach others to do what I can do, it can't be just magic... and if these teachable gifts are in the Bible, then it has been teachable for over two thousand years.

Constance continually strives to advance her knowledge and is currently in the process of attaining her Ph.D. and DOCTORATE in Natural and Integrative Medicine.

ALSO AVAILABLE

Play the game *Ikona* – Discover Your Inner Genie

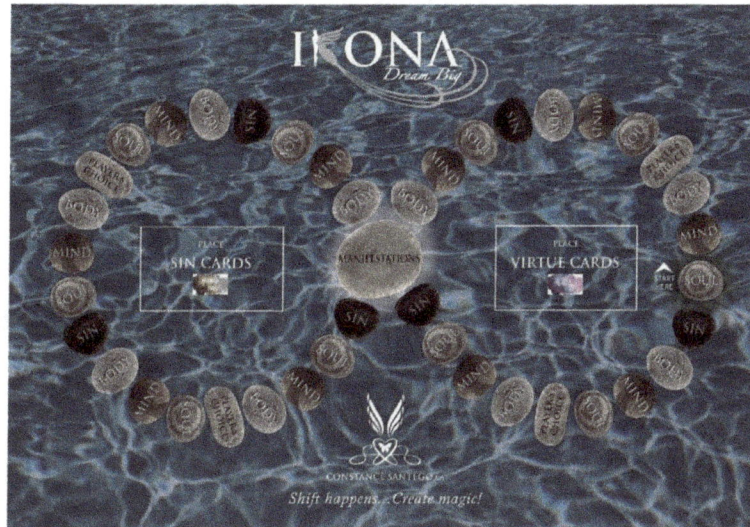

For additional information on

Constance Santego's

wide range of Motivational Products, Coaching Sessions, Spiritual Retreats,
Live Events and Educational Programs

Go to

www.ConstanceSantego.ca

Follow on Instagram - Constance_Santego and
Facebook - constancesantegoo

Subscribe and receive Free Information and Meditations on my
YouTube Channel - Constance Santego

www.ingramcontent.com/pod-product-compliance
Lightning Source LLC
Chambersburg PA
CBHW080621030426
42336CB00018B/3033